The F Word

Confessions of a Cheesecake Lover

Small Changes for Extraordinary Results Using Keto and Low Carb

Emma Martin

First published by Ultimate World Publishing 2021
Copyright © 2021 Emma Martin

ISBN

Paperback: 978-1-922597-12-0
Ebook: 978-1-922597-13-7

Cover design: Ultimate World Publishing
Layout and typesetting: Ultimate World Publishing
Editor: Isabelle Russell
Cover photography © Chay Doleman

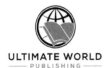

Ultimate World Publishing
Diamond Creek,
Victoria Australia 3089
www.writeabook.com.au

Testimonials

'A fantastic read for anyone, especially those looking to get off the sugar/carb speed-train we unwittingly board due to popular misinformation. Emma explains the history and science that has led to this mass embarkation in an easy to read, humorous and heartfelt way.'

Cherie Farley,
Business Owner and Mum of four girls

'There is a difference between theory and experience. Emma has clearly experienced the benefits of a ketogenic lifestyle that have motivated her to do the deep work in order to understand the history and the science. This is a deep dive that will challenge much of the modern nutritional paradigm as well as our deep-seated biases. I couldn't recommend it more.'

Dr. Charles Brian Johnson BS Biomed Sci,
Doctor of Chiropractic (USA) Dipl. Acupuncture
(AACA) Fellow of F.A.A.C.A., C.C.A.c.

'This book is an easy read and very logical. It opened my eyes to know how move forward and, so far, it has helped me lose 2.8 kilograms. I'm going to continue to share it with my daughter to educate her on how to help her brain in the process. Thank you, Emma, you have opened my eyes on how easy it is to get back the energy I had.'

Carolyn Robinson,
Proud Mum

'What a fabulous, engaging read, full of personal stories and speckled with humour. Although I knew much of the medical stories relating to fat, keto and sugar, seeing them laid out before me was absorbing and at times frustrating and confronting. I've recently commenced my keto voyage and I am loving it. Thank you, Emma, for sharing your learning, insights and results, and for providing encouragement to others to embrace the change and to challenge what we are led to believe. Looking forward to trying some of the recipes, especially the cheesecake.'

Kay Thorn,
Communications Supervisor,
Queensland Fire and Emergency Services

'I love how Emma has taken a complex subject and broken it down in a way that is very easy to understand. Her ability to reference her own experiences and stories and back them up with science makes for very easy reading. If you have been confused by what you should/should not be eating. Please read this book—it will change your life!'

Andrew Johnson,
Health Coach

'I picked up this book because I have been a believer that the keto diet is the way to a healthier life, but sometimes it is difficult to know where and how to start that journey... this book gives you the knowledge and the tools to take action and make some noticeable yet easy changes in your lifestyle. I now feel confident that I can do this keto health change armed with the true facts and the recipes that the book offers me. Thanks, Emma.'

Chantal Robert, Business Owner and Mum

'I totally enjoyed Emma's rendition of the history of the way we eat. I was fascinated at the depth and detail she uncovered about the scientists and researchers that have moulded the standard diet most people follow and believe to be the way we should eat. It is refreshing to find there is an alternative and a way to break the cycle many of us are caught up in. I especially enjoyed the way Emma has woven her childhood throughout her revelations, it truly makes me feel confident I can beat the crazy diet cycle.'

Ruth McMullan,
Registered Nurse

'Well-researched and very informative for anyone wanting to start a keto diet.'

Susie Pitt,
Holistic Nutritional Practitioner and Educator

'Emma's book is fabulous! It is an inspiration and great help for anyone who wants to improve their health and enjoy the most delicious food on Earth! An absolute *must* on everyone's bookshelf!'

Gabriella Kispal,
Functional Medicine and Keto Practitioner

'Great read—Emma is able to explain scientific information in a way that is easy to understand and entertaining at the same time. I have started to make some of the small changes recommended in the book and am already seeing results, I am sleeping a lot better and have more energy. The best thing is I don't feel that I am on a diet.'

Peta Holton,
Teacher

'This book is a game changer for those who don't want to give up food they enjoy, with some little tweaks. This book will change your life.'

Wendy Hinschen,
Child Educator

'I loved this book. It made losing weight fun and learning how the body responds is so interesting. I'm inspired to start my journey, not only to lose weight, but to feel better and teach my body to respond better. I love how Emma candidly talks about how your life has led to this moment, and how your thought processes affect you. The recipes are great too! Love it, love it, love it.'

Kym Dallinger,
Mum

'Truly an inspirational book from beginning to end! Full of eye-opening and mind-blowing scientific facts and relatable to the everyday Australian woman! Absolutely *loved* it!

Charlotte Morgan,
Actor, Dancer and Inventor

Dedication

I would like to acknowledge our keto and low carb community, for being so generous in sharing of information and shining the light so brightly. A big shout-out to Joe Rogister and Kristy Walker, whose passion and enthusiasm are so very contagious, and insights are so very precious to me.

To my beautiful daughter, Hannah, you are my reason, my why. I want you to know that absolutely anything is possible if you believe and I'm excited to know that my passion for learning has rubbed off on you, and that you'll never have to ride the diet roundabout like I have. I love that we are friends and that our lines of communication and understanding are *always* open. I love you, bun.

Disclaimer: this book is not intended to replace any medical advice from your practitioner. If in doubt, always check with your healthcare provider.

Contents

Testimonials   iii

Dedication   vii

Introduction: Wobbly bits   1

Part 1. What, why and when... 13

Chapter 1: It wasn't the cheesecake   15

Chapter 2: You're not an island   21

Chapter 3: You've been told BS   43

Chapter 4: The big fat lie   61

Chapter 5: What the fat?   75

    A few friendly fat recipes   82

Chapter 6: Voldemort   87

Chapter 7: The goss on grain   103

Part 2. The how to.. 111

Chapter 8: The great undoing   113

Chapter 9: You are not a tree   121

Chapter 10: Hidden keys   129

Chapter 11: How do you eat an elephant?   139

Part 3. Level up... 149

Chapter 12: Unlocking the storage shed   151

Chapter 13: Dances with brooms   169

Chapter 14: There is no wagon   183

Afterward   187

Inspiring information   189

The recipe files..**193**

Keto pantry staples   195

Simple snacks   196

Simple sweets   206

Easy dinners   213

Superb sauces   225

Beautiful breads   228

Cheat sheets and quick reference guides   233

Appendix A   237

Appendix B   243

About the author   245

Resources and references   247

Testimonials (continued)   257

INTRODUCTION

Wobbly bits

'We are not designed to be chronically ill.'
PROFESSOR TIM NOAKES

A few years ago, I found a way of eating that set me free. I had been diligently following the low-fat diet recommended by the Government called 'the food pyramid'. I just couldn't shake the fog, the 'hangriness' or the food hunts. I had no willpower whatsoever and I'd re-promise myself almost *every day* that I'd lose the weight I'd gained. I was eating lean meat, veggies, plenty of fruit and grains, but I couldn't say no to the donuts. Apart from those irresistible donuts, and the occasional sneaky chocolate bar, I was pretty much following the food guidelines set out by the Australian Government. I cut the fat off my meat like they asked me to, I switched to low-fat options wherever I could, and I steered well clear of cream and full-fat dairy, even though I loved these and they satisfied me. I replaced butter with vegetable oil and ate the standard three meals a day plus snacks. Just like I was told to.

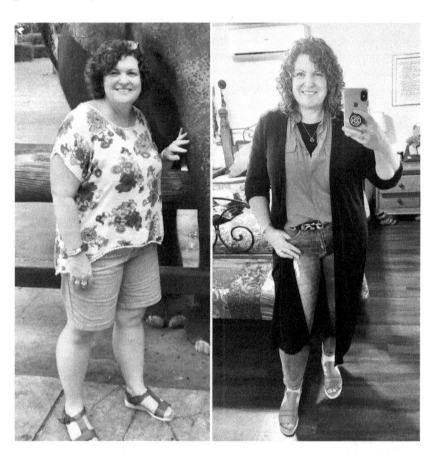

2018 vs. 2021

But I was struggling. I was moody and restless, my energy didn't last and I was always looking for the next snack. I was bloated, tired, impatient and my pants were like what my grandmothers had worn in their seventies—stretchy waisted with baggy shirts covering my wobbly bits. I like to call this 'cheesecake' because that's where consumed goodies landed on my body.

I have fallen off every 'diet' I've ever tried. I have constantly felt like I was failing, and I was a regular at self-torture and the guilt cycle. I share this with you, so you know that I *feel* you. If you don't share these challenges, but struggle with your mood, energy and sleep, then at the very least, you have a sense of where I'm coming from. Maybe you're skinny-fat—you look awesome and fabulous on the outside, but you struggle with impulsivity, succumbing to cravings, and lack of clarity and focus.

Please note that this is *not* a diet book; it's a collection of hints, tips, strategies and recipes to help *you* never fall off another one of *those* 'D-words'. I want to pay it forward and teach you what was taught to me—what I did that helped me shed four jeans' sizes in just months (actually only 13 kilograms—more on that later). I reclaimed my brain and got off the crave coaster. When people had said '*it's a lifestyle, not a diet*' to me a few years before, I was the one who rolled my eyes. I just went *pfffft* at them—*whatevzzzzz*…. It sounds incredibly cheesy to say this, but I finally found my forever. I feel ridiculously better, and I would love you to experience this, too. This has prompted me to write this book, and expel some of the diet myths and lies you've been fed.

When I found this freaking amazing way of eating—rich sauces, butter, cream in my coffee, eating the skin on the roast chicken and even the fat off lamb chops—I couldn't believe it.

How on earth could this impact my weight so quickly, as well as offer substantial health improvements, and that of my family's health too, so dramatically?

At first, I upped my fats *very* cautiously and sceptically, and lowered my carbs, sugar and processed foods little by little. I remember saying to my partner over a breakfast of eggs benedict (because I could), that if this *didn't* work, I'd be the size of a house. Actually, that day I didn't finish the sourdough bread that the poached eggs were sitting upon, as I would have previously. I was full and satisfied, not still hungry, like I'd been for the past 20 years.

In reality, this kinda *had* to work. I was 47, getting rounder, especially around my tummy area, and I knew I'd be fighting menopause hormones very soon, which would make it more difficult to reduce the number on the scales. What I didn't know at the time was that I had become *insulin resistant*, my body locked in fat storage mode.

As I made these little changes, not only did the weight fall off around my tummy, face and feet—is there a better reason to go shoe shopping?!—I also started to feel *so* much better. The brain fog (that I didn't even know I had) cleared, my thoughts had space, my bloating subsided, my mood lifted, and my energy dramatically improved. I was *bouncing* out of bed and I wasn't constantly on the food hunt. The pantry raids stopped. I didn't yell at my daughter, and I was a calmer mum. Best of all, as a family, we saved *so* much money. It really seemed too good to be true. I was *waiting* for the 'fail', but it didn't come.

At first, I thought it must have been a placebo—as in, I expected it to work, so it did. But it *wasn't* my imagination. I felt so good, and I started shouting about it! This success compelled me to share my experience *very* loudly, as those who know me can attest to. Sorry, not sorry. Friends and family who came along for the ride, saw success too, so I knew it wasn't just my imagination.

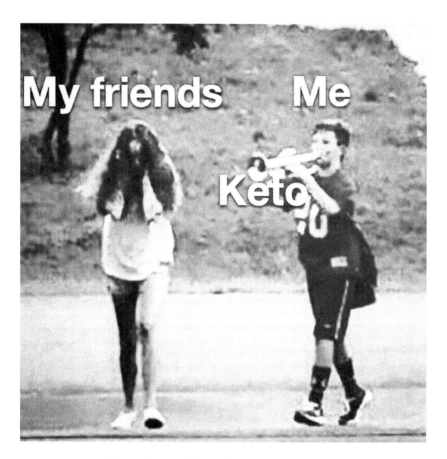

**Me, when I first found keto. Who
am I kidding… it's still me.**

My friend, Leanne, was one of the first to come along on this
journey. She had been struggling and although not overweight,
she just didn't feel comfortable. She was really despressed and
locked in sadness mode. Within a few days, as I coached her,
she saw her mood improve and started to leave her house again
and take part in the activities she enjoyed, like bushwalking and
going to the beach. Seeing her joy made me resolved to share
even more passionately.

My friends were seeing similar results and some, for the first time in their lives, weren't slaves to food anymore. Their ability to cope with their kids and partner increased, their fog lifted, and their sleep improved.

I started questioning and delving into the food pyramid we'd been told to follow since the 1970s, and what I discovered through my digging was that this dogma was based on completely *unsubstantiated* research.

Heads up—I'm not a doctor. I'm not a nurse or a practitioner, I'm not a scientific researcher. I'm somebody who became *extremely* passionate about this lifestyle and was shown where to find the information. I learned how to read PubMed documents and dug deeper to find out why on earth we got to this place as a human race, and why we are getting sicker and fatter. I learned and I researched, then I learned some more. I now hold a Diploma of Nutrition, because I needed to educate myself on the facts. This led me to complete a certified Keto Coach course, mostly because I wanted to better understand why the heck this works, but also to be able to coach others with the *correct* information. Many of my coaching customers have seen unbelievable results, *just* using really simple switches. Crazy.

You should always check with your doctor, however—a word of warning—they do not always understand. I urge you to keep looking till you find one who does. Doctors who share this lifestyle are increasing day by day, however the ones in your neighbourhood will possibly not be yelling thorough the rooftops because it's dangerous for your medical licence to do that in our current health climate.

> ## 'Science evolves by being challenged, not by being followed.'
> DR. GARY FETTKE

Dr Gary Fettke is a Tasmanian orthopaedic surgeon who was reprimanded and silenced by the Australian Health Practitioner Regulation Agency (AHPRA), stating he was he not qualified to give nutritional advice, for suggesting patients eat low-carb diets. Dr Fettke became passionate about nutrition after amputating limbs of diabetic patients whose diets were a tremendous contributor to the problem.

One of his patients, Julian Robinson, who had to have his leg amputated because of complications from diabetes, said the diet changed his life for the better. Yet an anonymous complaint from a dietician at the hospital where Fettke practised, sparked an investigation by AHPRA.

It was ruled that he was working *'outside his scope of practise and he was not qualified to give specific nutritional advice'*. He was ordered to stop speaking about the low carbohydrate, high fat diet. But Dr Fettke refused to be silenced.

Knowing that as a result, he could lose his medical license, Dr. Fettke made the decision to continue to give out empowering nutritional advice *'as a matter of principle'* and eventually received an apology. Two-and-a-half years later, AHPRA repealed its decision completely and cleared Dr Fettke of all charges.

He also received a written apology: *'There is no harm in Gary, nor any other health professional in Australia, recommending Low Carb Healthy Fat principles...'*

In another example, in 2014, Professor Tim Noakes was reported to the Health Professions Council of South Africa for giving 'unprofessional' dietary advice. He was advocating a low-carb, high-fat diet… in a tweet. He also had *reversed* the patient's diabetes, but because it was in contrast to government recommendations, what followed was a four-year legal process of mammoth proportions.

I met Kerry and her family a few months ago at my market keto stall. She was a bit of a mess, actually. Her family were on the verge of falling off the health precipice, and she was only just holding it together.

Her husband had been told that if he didn't do something immediately to change his path, he'd be very soon an insulin-dependent diabetic. When I met her, she was so eager to change her family's health, that she got busy learning, making small sustainable changes and has made some incredible headway.

She says, *'Amazing start for us. Nine kilograms in eight weeks. Our whole adult family. We changed our doctor to one that understands this lifestyle. My hubby who is diabetic went from BS16 (blood sugar) to normal in a few short months and is down to just 1/4 of his medication for D2. Woohoo!'* He has reversed his diabetes 2 in under three months using keto and low carb. Pretty exciting and crazy hey?

How on earth did we get here?

The last 60 years in nutrition science paint a pretty terrible picture. The short version is that scientists responded to an ever-growing number of heart disease cases which skyrocketed between 1900 to 1950 and led to the hypothesis that fat in our diets was to blame, despite us having existed on that, since the Palaeolithic era. The inconclusive blame on dietary fat, due to its 'effect on cholesterol', was touted as a universal truth even *before* it was proven. The big public health bodies adopted this hypothesis, and it became 'law'.

There have been many vocal doctors and scientists over the years, like Tim who have dispelled the myth that 'fat makes you fat', however they have been quickly silenced into submission, research grants disabled, and voices ridiculed.

Among some of the more vocal campaigners were Dr John Yudkin, the British nutritionist who suffered the wrath of opponent Ancel Keys (more on him later), Vilhhjalmur Stefansson, a 1900s anthropologist who lived with the Inuit eskimos and existed mainly on fat for over a year, and George V Mann, a professor of biochemistry who studied the dairy and meat-loving Maasai in Kenya and Tanzania, through to vocal champions today, like Dr Jason Fung, Dr Paul Mason and journalist authors, Nina Teicholts and Gary Taubes.

These people are well-respected and have taken time to look for gaps in the evidence. I'm asking for your open mind because this book will possibly contradict your current beliefs.

What if the food pyramid is wrong *and* these scientists, doctors and researchers are *right?*

If your goal reading this book is simply to be told the answer to the question, 'What can I do to remain a healthy weight or lose the excess fat I have?', the answer is this: stay away from preservatives, and carbohydrate/sugar-rich foods, such as beer, fruit juice and soft drinks, pastries, grains and sweets. The sweeter the food, the easier it is to over-consume and the more 'cheesecake' you'll store, most likely damaging your brain in the process.

We are going to take a look in this book at why this is so and, shortly after, take some small steps for extraordinary results.

Mmmm... Cheesecake

My very favourite treat in the chiller cabinet at a café is baked New York cheesecake. I love the brown caramelised crust that melts in my mouth, the creamy texture of the cheesecake and the crumbly biscuit base. I love that it's sweet, but not too sweet, and soft and silky in the middle. Eating it used to make me feel *sooooo* guilty. Plus, my body loved to bank it around my middle. I have since found a guilt-free recipe for this—you'll find this and many others in the recipes section of this book.

I've shared lots of very simple, easy-to-make, yummy meals and desserts (including the cheesecake on the cover), along with cheat sheets and swap guides. Most of these I can't take credit for—they were shared with me when I stumbled headlong into this lifestyle and now, I'm paying it forward and sharing them with you. This knowledge took me off the craving train, melted the fat off my belly, lit up my brain and healed my love-hate relationship with food. I love food. I hate that I craved it and had no control, but by using these tips, it wasn't hard to heal that relationship.

Did I mention I have since been able to enjoy the yummiest food ever?

We are going to teach your body to eat its own fat—to do what it is supposed to do—and how to tempt your own metabolism into burning those fat stores for amazing energy, the best mood, the clearest focus, less food slavery and cravings, the most amazing sleep, great feelings of fullness and the happiest brain you can possibly imagine.

If that sounds good to you, then read on.

PART 1.

What, why and when...

CHAPTER 1

It wasn't the cheesecake

'*Comparison is the thief of joy.*'
PRESIDENT THEODORE ROOSEVELT

Even as a little girl, I remember feeling fat. I probably wasn't, I was probably just a bit chubby at a few points in my youth.

The point is, that I always *thought* I was tubby. My mum used to say she hoped my 'growth spurt' would end on the up, not the out. Ouch. I remember not feeling worthy based on my perceived chubbiness and stockiness. I'm 5'4, so a little extra me goes a long way, dang it. I only ever need a few extra kilos to turn my body into an apple shape, with cheesecake around my middle and little legs sticking out the bottom. Even today, but especially back then, I compared myself to my friends, my stepsisters, and even people I didn't know, based on what I *thought* I saw in the mirror. I know now, this flawed perception of myself was based on a stacking of events, seemingly innocent and well-meaning comments from influential people in my life, perceived evidence, swinging emotions and a filing cabinet filled with 'proof'. I'd built up this crazy idea that I wasn't good enough, skinny enough or tanned enough, yet somehow lost sight of the fact that I was fun, passionate, excitable, reasonably intelligent and worthy of love.

Perspective

My early years were spent in a beautiful and fertile part of the Queensland hinterland in Australia. I lived with both my parents and my brother in a small house made of weatherboard, timber floors, and a corrugated iron roof that you could hear the rain on. There was a light and bright sunroom with straw-coloured seagrass matting on the floor where the cats used to laze in the sun. I remember the smell of the bush—yesterday, today, tomorrow, with its bright green foliage and lilac floral fragrance, wafting through the slotted glass louvre windows on sunny summer afternoons.

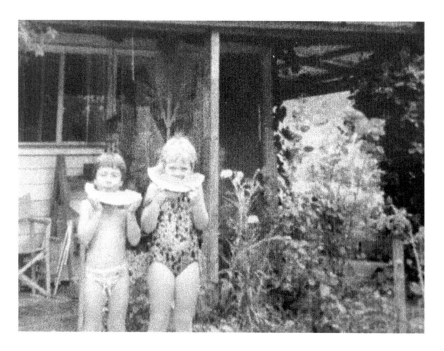

When watermelon smiles back at you!

We lived on a few hectares of land. We had trees to climb and a stream at the back of the property with mossy slippery rocks. The *really* big rock we called Chief Sitting Rock. This bears no relevance to the topic of my book whatsoever, I just wanted to give you a snapshot of my childhood. It was a happy one. We used to spend hours down the creek, catching frogs and tadpoles, throwing moss at each other and playing inventive kid type games. Dad built a downhill flying fox with a sturdy rope that ran from the big, forked tree just below the house, all the way to the bottom of the hill. It had a horizontal bar to hold on to and it was terrific fun, hanging on for grim life, as we slid down the rope to the bottom—putting aside the rope burn and skinned knees. We were pretty active as kids.

We had a mischievous white goat called Scruffy who regularly escaped and ate Mum's garden, we collected fresh eggs from our chooks and tended to the healthy green veggie patch. We collected fresh milk in urns from Mrs Rudd up the road and skimmed the cream straight from the top. When mum wasn't watching, I'd shovel a spoonful of it right into my mouth and relish the silky texture. We got seasonal produce from the local markets, farms or little shop down the local main street. We weren't affluent—sometimes we really struggled, but we always had a roof over our head and enough fresh food to eat.

My mum is a keen and knowledgeable gardener. She taught me about plants, organic gardening, and to this day, has a passion for unusual and healing herbs. It was rare for us to eat packaged and processed foods, as she had trained as an occupational therapist and gained knowledge of the body and nutrition.

For our main meal at night, we ate mostly meat, and vegetables from our garden. Our meals were, from what I remember, quite often padded out with potato. A good filling staple, I guess. I remember Mum buying whole sides of lamb, for economy mainly, so she used to get pretty creative, finding one thousand and one different ways to cook the same meat, and I guess this has rubbed off on me too. She was (and still is) a pretty amazing and resourceful cook. I also remember her doing a Cordon Bleu cooking course, so between all these factors, our food was both delicious and nutritious. I didn't actually realise this was my childhood snapshot until I started writing about it. How blessed was I?

For breakfast, my brother and I had toast with Vegemite or home-made marmalade, or cereals called Nutri-Grain or Weetbix (makes for healthy kids, right?) with milk and honey, and a vegemite sandwich in our lunchboxes, probably like most Aussie kids. We were 'allowed' lunch from the school canteen once a week and it was always a sweet, flavoured milk and some kind of sausage roll, pie, or sandwich and a piece of fruit.

We ate *real* butter. Always real, salted, yummy. I remember my Pop plastering his morning toast with *slabs* of butter and my grandmother nit-picking at him, like she always did. *'Like a little bit of toast with your butter?'* she would tease. Her words still echo in my mind years later, feeding guilt about something as natural and enjoyable as butter. She, too, believed the unsubstantiated lie about saturated fats—lies that say fats kill you, block your arteries and lead to nasty coronary heart disease.

There is *no*, and never was any, substantiated evidence to support this 'fat as a killer' theory. Not one iota. It was all based on manipulated correlations from cherry-picked data, not actual scientific evidence.

But we all believed it. We followed the dietary guidelines. We did as we were told. That flawed and unsubstantiated hypothesis was adopted willingly without evidence and is responsible for a truckload of the current health afflictions we are grappling with today. Issues like obesity, type 2 diabetes, heart disease, high blood pressure, stroke, dyslipidaemia, gallbladder disease, osteoarthritis, some cancers and tumours, sleep apnoea and breathing or asthma-related issues. Mental illnesses such as depression, anxiety and other brain function disorders including Alzheimer's and dementia are all on the rise and we currently treat them with medication, not through nutrition.

Few events in history have been as detrimental to the health of many as the food pyramid we've been following—a flawed study by the few, that became truth based on filtered incorrect information and followed by many. One dietary food group, that occurs naturally in nature, and by no coincidence, with a lot of our proteins, was blamed and made the scapegoat.

I met keto-caterer, Karissa, through our community, who had struggled with body image and mindset her whole adult life. She was previously a yo-yo dieter like I was, so we connected immediately. She received a devastating, but life-altering, phone call in March 2020 that didn't deliver the best of news—she was booked in for knee surgery and the local hospital said they couldn't complete the operation because her BMI was too high risk. Karissa was advised that she would need to have her surgery at a hospital with intensive care beds, rather than locally. She did have her surgery the next day, however she was devastated and embarrassed by this situation and began looking for answers, which led her to finding keto. She was supported by Dr Brian Johnson, a practitioner in Murwillumbah, who holds a Bachelor of Biomedical Science and six months later, she had not only melted an extraordinary 25 kilograms off her body, but regained her confidence, sleep, mood and clarity of thought. In November of 2020, Karissa was introduced to bio identical exogenous ketones by Dr Brian, and she was stunned at the difference in her energy levels—she describes ketones as a game-changer. Twelve months on, she has reached her goal size, has lost just over *36 kilos* and is vibrant and excited that she has been able to achieve a result like this using nutrition and mindset. She, too, as you can imagine, shares passionately.

The 'F word', if you haven't guessed already, is **FAT.**

CHAPTER 2

You're not an island

In this book I'm going to share some of those ridiculously simple changes you can make for extraordinary results. I can't stress enough that I wrote this book, to share with you, that if you've ever fallen off every diet and feel like a failure, *it's not your fault.*

So... just what if?

If the current government-recommended food pyramid we are following is correct, then *why* are we all getting fatter, sicker and struggling to stay healthy? If what we are following is correct, then why are the diseases I mentioned earlier on their way up, not down? Why is the developed worlds' health on a downhill slide?

What if the *very* food we've been told to eat more of, as *diet staples*— cereals with low-fat milk, fat-free dairy, refined grains, potatoes (hold the butter) and pasta, refined oils, feedlot meat—actually *reset* our physiology to sabotage all our best efforts.

What if, *just what if,* what we have been told is wrong?

The implication of this advice that we've been following is that if you eat too much and don't move enough, you get fatter. Thanks for the guilt cycle, Government! No more! You'll be happy to read that the hypotheses of *'calories in, calories out'* and *'eat less, move more'* are, in fact, incorrect and unfortunately ignore many factors like hormones, extraordinarily high consumption of over-processed seed (vegetable) oils, massive amounts of food that isn't food, preservatives, additives and higher stress levels, among other things. In an attempt to tackle the threat of many escalating diseases, much attention has incorrectly been paid to the number of *calories* present in food.

The terrible advice we have been given for the last seven decades, is that if you can't lose weight, you're fat and lazy and not trying hard enough.

Have a think though. Why would Big Pharma want you off your meds? Why would Big Food want you to stop buying consumables in pretty packaged boxes? It's a profitable business.

We live in an era where doctors prescribe medications, as they have been taught to do at medical school, instead of identifying and healing the cause. I'm not bagging the doctors; I'm just suggesting that it's possible most don't understand nutrition. Did you know that the average doctor completes just one hour of nutrition training at medical school? If you want to lose weight, the advice we're given by our well-meaning doctor is to eat less and move more. It's simply not true. Both the young, open-minded doctor Kerry and her family are working with, and Dr Brian, the keto doc, understand that nutrition is at the root of most illness and are willing to look at the cause to reverse symptoms, rather than the other way around. They understand that things like hormones, sleep, gut microbiota and stress *also* impact our waistlines, and that it's not all about 'calories in, calories out'.

I remember visiting a doctor seven or eight years ago, asking what I could to do lose the excess fat I was carrying and wondering if the answer might lie with the contraceptive rod inserted into my left arm. Her reply: *'No, dear, it's what you're stuffing in your face.'* She continued to advise me to 'eat less, move more' with no practical follow-up advice or any tips whatsoever. Needless to say, that advice wasn't particularly effective, and I didn't return to her because I felt pretty bad about myself and even more like a failure. I now know the answer lay with balancing hormones, specifically insulin.

Today, I coached a client of mine who had been given this *exact same advice*. No wonder we are confused. Doctors talk of patients becoming more insulin resistant and see ever-increasing numbers of obesity and chronic lifestyle-related conditions. So, they do as they have been trained. They prescribe. Recently, I was at a conference, listening to world thought leader, Dr Ken Ford, speak about emerging scientific evidence around the metabolic state of ketosis, who said, *'If your GP still believes in 'energy in, energy out', it's time to find a new GP.'*

Cardiac surgeon, Dr Phillip Ovadia says *'If your doctor isn't interested in treating your issue with diet and lifestyle, you may like to reassess your doctor'*. Bam!

You don't need surgery, pills or crazy gym workouts to help you burn your stored fat—you just need to make small adjustments to your diet and throw in a little movement. Truly.

So, breathe, and know you're not alone. We can fix this. *Tiny* changes like switching from skim milk to cream in your coffee can yield massive health benefits, a smaller waistline, and a clearer brain in the process. I know right. Crazy. And no, cream won't make you fat.

Ingrained beliefs

I was lucky enough to grow up close to my grandparents. On some school holidays we would stay with them on the sunny canals of Mooloolaba on the Sunshine Coast. My grandparents purchased the land in the early seventies. It was in the middle of nowhere at the time and Mooloolaba was a sleepy little one street, beachside town. It cost them a small fortune, but it was right on the water and my Pop loved to fish and catch mud crabs. It was pretty idyllic— summer days in the warm Australian sun, swimming in the sub-tropical waters, fishing for shiny bream and sand-loving flathead off the bessa brick wall.

My favourite part was always in the afternoons, when we'd walk to the beach with my dad's mum. We called her Mardi, a name she'd chosen because she didn't love the idea of being named like a grandma. I liked the beach, but the best bit was when we'd visit the little local ice-cream shop with the colourful red and white awnings on the way home. We'd peer over the counter and try to choose an ice-cream flavour. To this day, the taste (or even the thought) of ice-cream in my mouth brings me back to this moment and the joy associated with it—Pavlov's dog.

Ivan Pavlov ran experiments in which he measured the salivation of dogs who were anticipating food. He experimented with bells, doors and tones signalling to the animals that food was coming. By way of association, Pavlov found that just the stimuli of these events could set off salivation and anticipation in the dogs. The same runs true for us and our memories of food.

We didn't really have many desserts growing up—we couldn't really afford them, and Mum didn't think they were necessary. Sometimes, when we went to my grandparents' place for dinner, we'd be allowed to have dessert, but only after we'd finished everything on our plates. At dinnertime, we weren't allowed to leave the table until we'd eaten it all. There was always a pile of peas (I'm not a fan) that found their way somehow from my plate to under the dinner table because if they were still on my plate, I'd be at this table still today. I've never forgiven the cats for not eating them for me!

A lot of you will resonate with the 'finish everything on your plate' rule. I suppose this was a belief that was passed down from our wartime grandparents from when food actually *was* scarce and they didn't know what, or when, the next meal would be. This has left me with an ingrained belief as an adult that I *must* eat all the food on my plate, or I would be wasteful.

We build associations with certain types of food as they activate the pleasure centre (dopamine) in the brain, like Pavlov's dogs. For me, the memory of those summer afternoons and ice-cream, is one of being loved. The thought of an ice-cream still activates that feeling of joy I felt on those sunny afternoons; like everything was right in the world.

These days, when I approach the restaurant in an Ikea store, the smell of vanilla triggers the same memories and feelings. Peter Alexander, the pyjama store, has this same smell trigger for me— one sniff of the sweet vanilla and they own me.

Maybe you have had pivotal moments like these too? Before I adopted this new lifestyle, I'd never been able to pinpoint my emotional attachments to food. I knew I had them but couldn't identify where or what they were. The more I learned inside our keto and low-carb community, the more I understood just how to recognise and deal with these emotional attachments to food triggers that had previously left me questioning my willpower, leading to a sense of failure and guilt.

At kindergarten, I remember hearing my (very brave) teacher saying to my mum that she thought I needed more love. She made this statement based on her observation that I wanted more of the baked goodies than the others, always asking for seconds. It makes sense to me now, as I guess those cakes were symbolic to me of what I had deemed to be love and affection, because of the feelings they evoked in me.

My parents divorced when I was eight. My dad moved away, and we saw him every second weekend. This was a pretty traumatic time for me, as I was really close to my dad, and I felt like he didn't care and had abandoned me. It's difficult to write about this even now, as in my eyes, he moved on with his own life, leaving me behind. When he eventually re-married, as a teen I managed to compare myself to my tanned, popular stepsisters (who I love) and I fell into a hole of comparison. These feelings of abandonment led to me using food as a crutch and solace for my emotions. Food comforted me. I didn't realise how impactful this had been in my own self esteem journey until it was raised by a mentor of mine recently.

Adulting

I left home for university at the tender age of almost 17 and discovered McDonald's for the first time. It was easy, cheap and tasty and I quickly developed a love affair with junk food. While at university, I was body-shamed, which only added to the food and image issues I had already gathered through childhood. I continued to eat my feelings, and the guilt at my lack of willpower was a constant companion.

As poor university students, we lived on a quality diet of cheap alcohol (anyone remember the three-dollar bottles of alcoholic Passion Pop? Basically, sugar in a bottle), McDonald's and student-style cooking, which looks a lot like reconstituted packets of two-minute noodles (cheap), toast with margarine and Vegemite (also cheap), mince (ground beef) and pasta or rice (also cheap and filling). For a treat, we'd buy a custard packet mix and have it with packet jelly (cheap). As you can see, a perfectly respectable well-balanced nutritious diet. Not.

The crazy thing looking back is that, at that time, I actually was a size 10–12—weighing approximately 65 kilograms and pretty darn healthy and active enough. Since then, I've yoyo'd with my weight over and over again. I just couldn't find the key. By my twenties and thirties, I'd made a few changes and was eating what the food pyramid suggested we eat. The Australian Dietary Guidelines suggested 6–11 serves of breads, grains and pasta, 2–3 serves of fruit and 3–5 serves of vegetables, 1–2 serves of low-fat dairy, lean meats, chicken and fish and eggs a day. Sugar, fats and oils were a 'sometimes food' at the top of the pyramid.

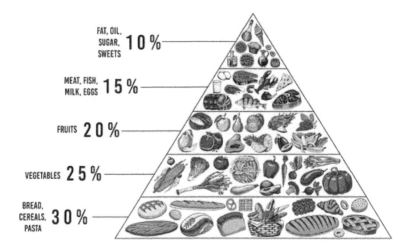

The food pyramid introduced to us c1980's

I started Weight Watchers when my daughter Hannah was a six-month-old baby in a pram in an attempt to lose the additional 15 kilograms worth of 'cheesecake' I'd managed to store during my pregnancy. My pregnant body had demanded macaroni cheese, while I was pregnant. At the time, a work colleague also commented, '*Jeez, you're stacking it on aren't you*', reinforcing those feelings of guilt and self-loathing about how much willpower I *didn't* have.

Now I know that if I'd eaten quality fats to fill me up, I wouldn't have been so ravenously hungry and making quick energy choices that sent my insulin (fat storage system) into overdrive. I managed to lose some of my accumulated baby fat by meticulously tracking all my food to points values daily, hourly and I almost reached my 'goal weight' a few times but I was *always* hungry, and fell off, making 'bad' choices. I wonder how many of you can relate to this.

I couldn't shake the weight permanently with Weight Watchers. Up and down, again and again, on and off, a period of 13 years. I loved their community though, and at one time found myself thinking maybe I'd be a leader sometime, but I kept falling off, so I wasn't a very good example.

The fat came back more persistently than ever, with *more* of its friends in tow, for a fat party where everyone was invited and there it stayed for years. I tried and failed at shakes, Weight Watchers (again), pills, Weight Watchers (yet again), coffee and cigarettes, low-fat—you name it, I tried it. I had resigned myself to forever wearing stretchy-waisted pants. The fact that I was now considering myself 'middle-aged' granted me some kind of acceptance, that I was destined to be round forever and that it was my lot to be chubby in life.

I now know that all these events in my youth and adolescence, were the beginning of my love affair with sugar and refined carbs, and my love hate relationship with food. I have finally learned why I constantly craved, without knowing why.

Did you know that sugar is *more addictive* than cocaine? And that starchy carbs like potato and pasta are processed the same way as sugar inside our bodies? It's not quite that simple, but you get the gist. Now I know that these foods activated a set of chemical reactions that played on the rewards centre in my brain.

Is it any wonder then, that this ultimately leads to the diet/fall off cycle that many of you will be so familiar with? It also, as a fabulous, unexpected bonus, reinforced my constant feelings of unworthiness and low self-esteem and failure.

And then, hallelujah. The light at the end of the tunnel.

I stumbled on keto/low-carb plus natural ketones a few years ago. The ketones cut my cravings and the food was delicious, filling and easy! It also went *against* everything I'd ever read. I regained my energy, conquered my cravings and dropped from a size 18 in those stretchy pants to a size 11 in fitted jeans, without exercise, in just 21 weeks and I have been able to maintain that almost effortlessly ever since.

It seemed extreme to me, to try something so radical as eating fat to lose fat, but I kid you not, even a few weeks in, it felt like a godsend. My brain worked, I started sleeping amazingly well, and I didn't have the nasty cravings. The freedom from food slavery and hunger was life changing. The energy I gained, lasted all day and I became more patient and much kinder, instead of being the raving hangry banshee I'd previously been. I think if I'd found this lifestyle a few years before, I'd have coped better with my ex-stepson, who was diagnosed with ADHD and asperges at the age of 12, although too late to save the relationship that had been broken, partly due to my inability to cope with stress. He and his dad adopted keto a year before I did and he had actually been telling me I should try it, to my previously deaf ears – because it seemed too hard at the time. They had adopted keto because being in ketosis is beneficial to the ADHD and autistic brain, due to neural connection pathway benefits. It was originally used over one hundred years ago to treat children with epilepsy and calm their brain.

This discovery of keto, although new to me, is not a new one, and it has led me to write this book and share the amazing results I've had, and sustained, with you.

A catalyst for change

I was shocked when I saw this photo of myself and my family in Bali, Indonesia in 2018. I remember being so excited that we were getting our photo taken with a beautiful Asian elephant, who had

the gentlest brown eyes and longest eyelashes I've ever seen—
even *if* you include the popular TV show *Married at First Sight*. I
remember feeling *so* excited and grateful for the opportunity and
we pre-ordered *that* photo, as you do.

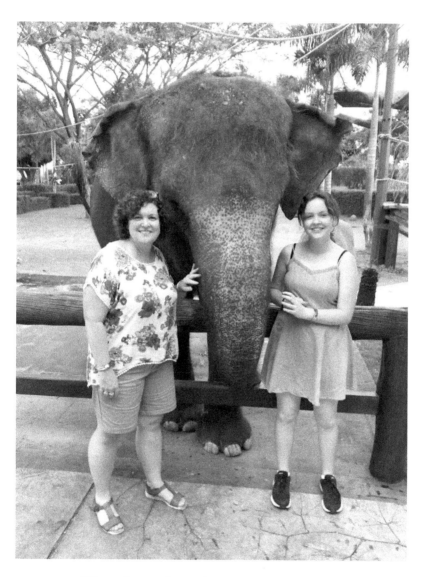

The photo that changed everything

When I saw this photo, my heart *sank*. I was gutted. I felt empty and ashamed. The person I saw looking back at me was a bloated, frumpy, middle-aged woman in stretchy-waisted pants who looked puffy and exhausted. The image I saw certainly did *not* match how I wanted to feel, and it *most certainly* wasn't the role model I'd pictured for my teenage daughter. Seeing that photo, I made a decision.

And that, is one of the most important things you can do for yourself. Decide. Then take action. Without both of these, you'll still be at the mercy of the whirlpool. Once you make a decision and commit, you'll be surprised how quickly you can impact your life.

I'd been watching a friend of mine and her weight loss journey for about six months. I knew she was spending time in nutritional ketosis (I didn't really understand what that was) and I could see she was shrinking. Not only was she shrinking; she was *absolutely glowing*. Her eyes were bright and her skin was clear. She had a definite spring in her step and I had been watching her sceptically. She was talking very passionately about how she felt, exactly like my daughter's dad had.

I started to Google 'keto' and 'low-carb' and what I read (read: clickbait) made me believe I was going to die—Dr Google told me that it might kill me! All the evidence I'd found pointed to the fact that restricting carbohydrates made you sick and caused liver or kidney failure, *blah blah blah*.

How, then, was it possible that she looked so incredibly healthy if fat kills you? And why wasn't my daughter's dad dead from eating too much fat?

As I followed and researched this lifestyle, I noticed all keto'ers had the same healthy glow. It took me a while to realise that most of us didn't understand what *this* was, and that I'd have to dig a bit deeper for the science—And dig, I did. I stumbled on a podcast that featured Dr Jason Fung speaking about methods for treating people with type 2 diabetes, combining intermittent fasting and nutritional ketosis to achieve brilliant results. I didn't have diabetes as far as I knew, however, knowing what I know now, I probably had insulin resistance. More on insulin resistance later—it's one of the biggest keys to losing your cheesecake and loving your brain.

Dr Jason Fung is a world-leading Canadian nephrologist. He's a kidney man, in other words. His stories and research echoed what I'd been hearing my friend say. I dug some more and found the *Low-Carb MD* podcast and also Dr Eric Berg, Dr Timothy Noakes and young Australian doctor, Dr Paul Mason. I was amazed as they shared the results their patients were experiencing.

I made a *choice*. I began.

When I shared what I was planning with my doctor and my friends, they were convinced that I was going to end up with high blood pressure, damagingly high cholesterol and wipe out my liver and kidney functions. This just wasn't the case. It was in fact, the very opposite.

I found an energetic, passionate, generous community and worked with a local nutrition-focussed doctor who guided me and took my bloodwork and benchmarks. These people drip fed me information, science and tips—exactly what I'm sharing with you.

My most recent blood tests (12 pages of them) show not only that all my internal functions are better than ever—my cholesterol is also perfect, thyroid and kidney functions top notch, my liver is healthy, my iron, vitamin D, B12 and mineral levels are exactly where they need to be and my blood sugar levels are balanced. No more insulin resistance. No wonder my energy levels are off the charts. As we went through the test results together, my doctor said enthusiastically, *'If I am as healthy internally as you, at the age of 49, I'll be ecstatic.'*

I used natural bio-identical ketones (I've referenced the only bio-identical natural ketones currently available for you in the back of the book in appendix B). Using these consistently allowed me to drop a lot of my excess fat remarkably quickly, because they cut my cravings and hacked my body into ketosis (fat burning mode). I used the ketones to cut the sugar cravings and implemented eating more healthy fat, dropping my carbs a little and adding some intermittent fasting, and for the first time in my life, I finally understood that falling off every single diet previously was actually *not my fault*.

It was such a relief.

Within a few days, I started to feel better. My fog lifted. My brain cleared. My sleep got better. As I dropped sugar and refined carbohydrates and replaced them with healthy fats, I noticed my cravings were almost non-existent and within a few weeks the constant headaches that I'd been experiencing were gone. Even my eyesight improved!

I felt amazing! I couldn't believe how well my brain worked on ketones, and I bounced out of bed, instead of being groggy and sluggish when I woke up. My skin cleared up and my pants got loose. My appetite no longer ruled me, and I wasn't swinging off the pantry door looking for snacks at feed-o-clock. I wasn't at the mercy of my previously hangry temper and lack of willpower that had ruled my life for so long. This was different—it didn't feel like a diet to me. I was a much more patient mother, and less of a raving banshee. As I got excited and started yelling about how I was feeling, many of my family and friends came for the ride. They had similar results to me.

My sister-in-law saw her blood pressure improve and great fat loss around her tummy, my brother lost his belly, his second chin and regained his spark. He looks ten years younger. Lisa fits into one leg of her old pants! There are dozens and dozens of stories like this, about people—just like you.

Early in my journey, my community decided to get together for a BBQ in the park. Because I love food and positive people, (who doesn't, right) I said yes to attending. When it was announced that they were going paddle boarding, my (ample) stomach turned. I didn't want to stand up in front of everyone on a wobbly paddle board, that was determined to de-horse me while I attempted to balance my overweight bits. I fought the fear and went along anyway. I remember sitting on the wooden salt-stained benches holding my coffee (with cream), watching their glee at mastering the wobbly boards and beating myself up at the same time for not being able to find my brave.

As I drowned in the dismay and disgust for the way I looked, my ancestral brain was taking me back to all the memories that had made me feel not good enough and unworthy. This brain is the one that is designed to protect us. Its role is to keep us safe, so it banks the knowledge and turns them into fears.

I was the little girl left on the bench when the school sports teams were picked. I was the body-shamed teen at university. I was the little chubby girl on the end of the front row in school photos. This, of course, leads to another guilt-and-repeat cycle. Maybe even a sneaky clandestine donut fix. You know, I've never shared this with anyone, but I used to stand in front of the mirror and call myself a 'big fat toad'. I was always so disgusted by what I saw.

Please know that when you look in the mirror, you'll see both your own best friend, and your worst enemy.

I can happily report that today, while I still can't balance to save myself, I feel comfortable enough in my swimmers when I look in the mirror, to not let it ruin yet another day of my life. These days, despite a bit of cheesecake still sitting there, I look in the mirror and tell myself that I'm magnificent. And that I *freaking rock*.

Finding this lifestyle has made me very passionate and I would like to extend my hand to you and help you make some simple changes in your own life because not only can you transform your own health trajectory, you can also have massive impact on many of those you care about too.

If I can do it, you can too. I hope that you find this book inspiring and packed with plenty of easy to implement, helpful step-by-step tips. You're going to learn some incredibly healthful hacks, mindset tips, hear real science and, *most importantly*, how to get back on if (when) you fall off.

There are many amazing resources for you at the back of this book, and I know it will be tempting for you to race straight to those, please don't go there first—It's incredibly important that you understand why, and how we got here, because you're going to experience people who aren't enlightened. People who don't understand. Yes, even your doctor may fall into that category.

So, when you're finished with this book, please pass it on or gift someone a copy. You may just change their life too. This knowledge will be your secret armour. It will give you the belief to *know* you're not *only* doing something amazing for your long-term health but also taking steps to nurture your brain as you age. Not only can you maintain the new you on the outside, you can simultaneously bio-hack your brain to safeguard your mental future.

I can promise you that if you hang in there, you'll see your waistline get trimmer, your brain fog will lift, your pants will fall off as you walk (buy a belt), your mood will lift substantially, and your sleep will improve. You'll see your skin clear up and your attitude improve. You won't be as snappy at your family and the self confidence that went missing will start to return. As your self-confidence comes back, you may find the courage to leap into that big dream you've been thinking about. You may get a promotion at work. You might even see the road rage disappear. You'll make better and more impactful decisions because you have a much, much clearer, working brain.

But you've got to *keep going*. This is *not* a race. This is about your health and it's a marathon, not a sprint.

Mindset

If you've picked up this book, you're probably ready. However, if you aren't completely committed to this process, you won't do it.

Waiting for the 'perfect moment' is a form of procrastination. It will *never* be the perfect time. Start with what and where you're at and learn as you go. You can level up as you progress.

How you feel today is a direct result of choices you've made in the past. You can choose to move forward today, right here, right now, because what you believe is *everything*. Absolutely everything.

Your mindset is one of the most important factors in this whole game. When you know what you want, and you believe you can do it, and you know *who* you're doing it for, you can achieve it, if you take some steps and *do* the do.

Who and what are you doing this for?
Is it the 'you' who you lost somewhere along the way?
Is it so you can play with your children, grandchildren?
What will this mean as you get healthier and think more clearly?
How will this impact the people in your life?
And who are you role-modelling this for?

Today I'm so grateful that my daughter will never have to know what it feels to be on the diet roundabout, because of the little changes we've made as a family.

Do the voices in my head bother you?

What little voices are you hearing in your head that say *you can't?* You didn't. You wouldn't. You shouldn't.

These voices are hangovers from your past (the bit of your mind that is designed to keep you safe)—so make a decision to leave that behind—you are moving to your future, right here, right now.

Those voices are in the past. I want you to change them to the positive. Those voices don't belong in your future. Let's reframe them.

In the past I believed that

_____

_____

I now believe that

_____

_____

When I fall off, I know that it's not really permanent. I can get back on – this is important to me because

_____

_____

Set your expectations and goals - please don't make them all surrounding weight loss. Pick some goals that aren't weight related. What your mind sees, you can achieve. Everything is created twice—once in our mind and the next in reality.

Write down your goals. Note how these sample goals below are positive based, not focused on the negative. Next, write down how you will be impacted in the future. For example:

I *will* fit into my size 12 jeans again and *will* be able to tie my shoelaces without my belly getting in the way.

I will eat more nutritious foods so that I can see my skin improve and my brain fog clear. Once I have achieved this, I will sustain this lifestyle in the long-term to positively impact upon my brain health for years to come.

I *will* make sleep a priority. I will not use my phone after 9 pm and I will practise mindfulness or self-love before checking my phone in the morning. This will impact me in the future to become be more positive.

I *will* speak to myself kindly. I will tell myself that I love myself every single day and know that if I make a mistake, it's only a learning opportunity. In the future, I will forgive myself and move forward faster.

Next, I want you to speak your goals. Say them out loud. When your brain hears you, you are quite literally rewiring it, as cheesy as it feels to say them aloud. It has been scientifically *proven* that *what* your brain hears, you can achieve.

You may like to create a mini vision board of what this looks like to you. I regularly have pictures stuck to my fridge door or pinned on my whiteboard. Use a magnet, not glue, because you're allowed to change your goals whenever you like – you are not cemented in concrete. If your goals change, that's completely cool.

Some non-weight related goals might include:

- better sleep
- cooking at home
- taking measurements
- being kinder to yourself
- fitting into the pants you were previously comfortable in
- feeling better to play with your kids
- moving more
- finding sustained energy throughout the day
- eating to satiety—fewer cravings
- looking after your brain health
- ageing gracefully

We are going to make some small but incredibly sustainable changes towards *just feeling better*. As you start this journey, your body may resist. It's a life-protecting mechanism to ensure you survive, so just know that it may take some time to rewire your brain, before its automatic. Be kind to yourself and give it time.

So, let's do this. Decide that you're worth it. *You've got this.*

CHAPTER 3

You've been told BS

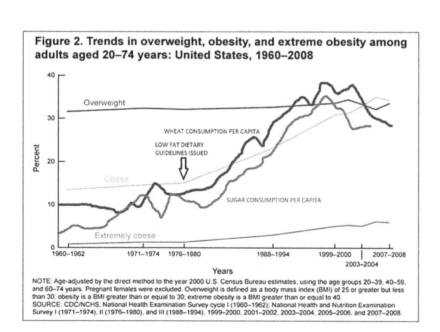

Figure 2. Trends in overweight, obesity, and extreme obesity among adults aged 20–74 years: United States, 1960–2008

NOTE: Age-adjusted by the direct method to the year 2000 U.S. Census Bureau estimates, using the age groups 20–39, 40–59, and 60–74 years. Pregnant females were excluded. Overweight is defined as a body mass index (BMI) of 25 or greater but less than 30; obesity is defined as a BMI greater than or equal to 30; extreme obesity is a BMI greater than or equal to 40.
SOURCE: CDC/NCHS, National Health Examination Survey cycle I (1960–1962); National Health and Nutrition Examination Survey I (1971–1974), II (1976–1980), and III (1988–1994), 1999–2000, 2001–2002, 2003–2004, 2005–2006, and 2007–2008.

Obesity rates start to climb from the late 70s, around the same time as the food pyramid was introduced.

Worldwide obesity has nearly tripled since 1975, not coincidentally, since the introduction of the current recommended eating guides.

According to the World Health Organisation (WHO), in 2016, more than 1.9 billion adults aged 18 years and older were overweight.

Of these, over a quarter were obese. These numbers have continued upwards in a worrying trend. Being obese increases your chances of metabolic illness and immune system dysfunction.

In 2018, the Australian National Health Survey showed that two thirds (67.0 per cent) of Australian adults were overweight or obese, representing an increase of 63.4 per cent from four years prior

Shockingly, 2018 statistics show that almost one quarter of our children are overweight or obese and the number is still rising.

The global snapshot isn't much better. In the UK, over 60 per cent of adults are overweight or obese and over 70 per cent in the United States of America.

Currently, 77 per cent of men and 53 per cent of women in the USA will either have diabetes or pre-diabetes by the end of 2021.

If these statistics shock you, they should. For years, we've been recommended that the fundamentally flawed policy of 'calories in, calories out' is the pathway to health.

We've been made to feel like gluttons if we can't control our greed for 'naughty' foods. We've been told that 'energy in equals energy out'. We are typecast as lazy and undisciplined if we don't work out at the gym every minute, when in fact, the information we have been given is *wrong*.

In order to understand why this isn't true, let's talk about our ancestors. Being metabolically flexible is *the only way* we survived as a species.

Our palaeolithic ancestors were generally carnivores. They may have lived in crude huts or caves. They hunted and foraged to eat and may have been lucky enough to gather some wild seasonal berries in summer. They ate whatever they could fish, catch, hunt, dig out of the ground or forage. Perhaps they would consume dairy from their herd. Some were nomadic, following the seasons, while others had settlements. Regardless of where or how they lived, they hunted and foraged for their next meal, often deprived of food for days at a time.

To their feast from a hunt, they may have added some root vegetables, nuts or berries. Every single bit of their catch was eaten, preserved or used, because food was precious and cost them energy to acquire. During the 'fed' times they would have eaten to satiety, made tasty, nutritious soup from bones (bone broth) and filled their food stores by preserving the excess. They survived due to being metabolically flexible (being able to change between using both native fuel sources—ketones and glucose)—and they thrived.

It's no coincidence that we, as humans seek out sweets. We are biologically wired to gather berries. Our survival depended on it. However, these berries weren't huge and juicy, and certainly weren't available all year round like they are today, in little plastic punnets, or frozen bags you can get from a door. When your body calls you to eat the sweet stuff, it's the ancestor kicking in. It compels you to 'eat to survive'—it wants you to grab that quick-burn fuel!

In Palaeolithic times, low blood sugar levels signalled 'it's time to eat', and it made perfect sense to consume berries—this was

Mother Nature's fastest way of restoring our normal blood glucose levels. On a biological level, hunger and sweet cravings made sure we wanted berries and sought them out.

When we use all of the glucose in our system, ketones are produced and our body uses stored fatty acids for fuel, instead of glucose. This is called ketosis and is a *survival mechanism* allowing access to a prime, clean fuel source that gives us supreme clarity, energy and focus.

Ketosis is a natural biological metabolic state that has ensured not only our survival, but also meant we thrived in times of scarce. In the absence of glucose from berries, carbohydrates (or donuts), we shift into ketosis and burn our 'cheesecake' for fuel. We weren't designed to store as much fat as we do, because it makes running after our meals rather challenging.

Ketosis is vitally important to humans. Our ancestors *needed* to be fuel-flexible. Ketosis gave them laser focus and stamina, not only to catch their dinner, but to subsist for long periods of time without food. Our ancestors most certainly didn't have a wonky-wheeled trolley that they could push into the back of someones ankles, through well stocked supermarket aisles, to hunt their food in fridges.

Anyone who has ever experienced nutritional ketosis will tell you that they feel superhuman. One of my mentors likes to say, *'I didn't know I had brain fog until it was gone.'* I have to remind myself that most humans in the well-fed western world haven't ever felt supersonic, because it seems so normal to me now, to have clear thoughts and great energy. I remember phoning my partner a few weeks into my journey, saying to him that I felt like I could run up the side a mountain—and I definitely don't run! The clarity of thought I felt and the fabulous energy on the day ketosis kicked in was a completely new experience for me. I'd never felt like that before! I became obsessed with how good I was feeling and was determined never to go back.

Another F-word: Feast

In paleo times, and even up until a few decades ago, we didn't have egg farms and battery hens, canola fields and orchards full of massive, juicy, genetically-modified oranges like we have today. I remember my grandmother talking about how she was excited to be gifted an orange as a Christmas present and how it was the best day of the year because of that orange. Incidentally, our fruit size has doubled in the last 50 years, thanks to commercialism, the need to feed the masses and to gain more profit and a competitive edge. The fruit we eat today is *fundamentally* different to what our ancestors would have foraged. Foods are bred to be larger, sweeter and juicier. Just like we have become.

Important turning points

In February 2021, a landmark decision was made by the Australian and New Zealand Ministerial Food Regulation Forum to reduce the five-star rating for fruit juice from five stars down to *two*. This is an *incredibly important* single step in the right direction because we are currently drinking our sugar.

Do you still believe that orange juice is a health food? In a whole piece of fruit, the sugar (fructose) is padded out with natural fibre that slows digestion into our blood stream. *This* is how nature intended us to consume natural sugars. When you remove fibre from fruit, there is *nothing* left to slow the blood sugar uptake in our body. This generates a massive flood of insulin, released by the pancreas, to clear the dangerously high levels of glucose from our blood. Insulin is the street sweeper of our body. If blood sugar is elevated for too long, damage occurs.

Popular beliefs, such as 'orange juice is good for us', have much to do with how well this was marketed to the world. Oranges are actually highly perishable, and with the invention of pasteurisation in the early 20th century, a juice boom followed. When the worldwide influenza outbreak occurred in 1918–1919 infecting thousands upon thousands (sound familiar?), juice popularity exploded. Understandably, people were suddenly very passionate about their health and with savvy marketing, fruit juice entered as the saviour. Ever since this, we've associated fruit juice with good health and sunny mornings, however the truth is a lot shadier. Commercial fruit juice is stripped of its fibre, freshness and nutritional benefits by industrial processing, and much of the flavour is artificially added back in. The result is a drink that's basically sugar in a glass—sugar that damages our natural metabolism and alters our immune system.

We eat food that isn't food. We import food from other countries when ours is out of season, laced with pesticides and preservatives. We modify crops to produce greater yields for greater profit. We process, strip and add vitamins back in that we have previously taken out. Madness.

To process sugars into our cells and muscles, even natural ones, including starchy carbs, (which are actually complex sugars), our bodies need insulin. And insulin, among other things, is a *fat storage hormone.*

I'll repeat that.

Insulin is a fat storage hormone.

48

If that is the *only* phrase you remember from this entire book, then my work here is done. This truly is the *single most important* key to your success. It's not about 'energy in equals energy out', even though that's what you've heard. It's actually about hormones like insulin (even if you're not diabetic), hormone balance, and growth factors that regulate our fat storage, and really not very much at all to do with calorie balance in the slightest.

Lost wisdom

My grandmother knew that fat didn't make you fat. She knew that starchy carb consumption made her body *hold on to*, and more importantly, *store* fat. This is certainly not a new message. Until the 1960s, this wisdom was conventionally accepted as truth. Carbohydrate-rich foods—bread, pasta, potatoes, sweets, beer— all the things we love, were seen to be fattening, and if you wanted to avoid being fat and feel great, you didn't eat them. Simple.

Our current food pyramid (the recommended intake of particular food groups) was introduced in 1978 and they suggested we eat 6–11 serves of carbohydrates a day. And so we did. Sales of this food group increased, while other food groups like meat and dairy declined, leading to the obesity epidemic and an unprecedented health crisis on a global scale.

One size does not fit all, however what we have learned, is that when we consume starchy carbs, our body releases insulin to process these complex sugars from our blood stream ASAP, to package them off into our muscles, liver and fat cells. The body contains approximately five litres of blood at any given time. In all of these 5 litres of blood, there is a tolerance for only 4 grams of sugar, that's less than a teaspoon! For our whole bloodstream!

Did you know that in a 250 millilitre glass of orange juice, there are 22 grams of sugar? That's a big blood sugar spike—over *five times* the amount our body can comfortably handle—just from a glass of 'health food'.

Enter insulin, dancing on in to clean up the excess rogue glucose (sugar) wandering around in the blood before it does too much damage. Excess sugar levels cause inflammation and are highly toxic.

Excess insulin secretion from our pancreas is caused by eating large amounts of easily accessible, energy-dense fast foods like our friend orange juice, refined carbohydrates like wheat flour, pasta and cereal grains, starchy foods like potatoes and rice, and sugars like high-fructose corn syrup (particularly damaging to the liver) and table sugar—these quite literally *make* us store fat, because of the insulin spike they create.

Insulin resistance

When we continuously spike our insulin, our pancreas and our cells become exhausted. This is the beginning of insulin resistance and it's the cause of many of the health afflictions that trouble our human race. We do not get fat because we overeat; we get fat because we consume carbohydrates (sugar) in excess. Hidden sugars in our packaged foods spike our blood sugar and raise our insulin.

Raise insulin, store fat. Repeat.

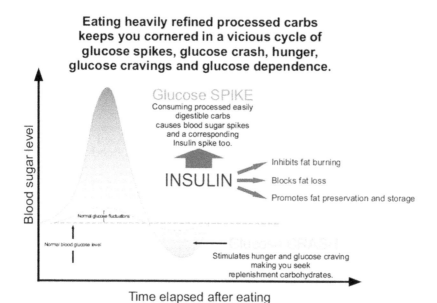

Eating heavily refined processed carbs keeps you cornered in a vicious cycle of glucose spikes, glucose crash, hunger, glucose cravings and glucose dependence.

Glucose SPIKE
Consuming processed easily digestible carbs causes blood sugar spikes and a corresponding Insulin spike too.

INSULIN → Inhibits fat burning

→ Blocks fat loss

→ Promotes fat preservation and storage

Normal glucose fluctuations

Normal blood glucose level

Stimulates hunger and glucose craving making you seek replenishment carbohydrates.

Blood sugar level

Time elapsed after eating

It's truly *that* important. Insulin is a *fat storage hormone*.

Dual fuelled

We have two fuel sources we can access for energy—glucose and fat. Glucose is stored in the liver and muscles, in handy little easy-to-access bundles called glycogen. These long-chain sugars are easy for our body to use quickly as instant energy. Reasonably important, wouldn't you say, to be able to access it quickly, if you had to escape from a predator?

Think of these little bundles of glucose as kindling for the fire and the quick fuel needed for survival. However, these fast access stores are limited. You can't fit many twigs in the basket. Once the stores of glucose are depleted, we use fatty acids and produce ketones to access our stored fat as an alternate sustainable energy source. Ketones

51

are only produced if glucose isn't present and allow us to unlock the 'cheesecake', that we didn't need during plentiful summer, and have been storing for survival in the winter, when food is scarce.

Our fat reserves are our long-term firewood stores, rather than the kindling that lights the fire and then burns out.

How many food-scarce winters have you experienced recently?

When we burn our own body fat, it's a very clean source of energy. If using glucose is the dirty coal engine, then energy from fat is clean solar power. Being able to burn body fat for energy means being able to activate the ancestral process our bodies were designed so efficiently for and to have the ability to flip between fuel sources. Most of us never experience this, as we are always refeeding and never accessing the metabolic switch.

In this plentiful age, we don't really have a short supply of energy sources. Big Food made sure of it. We have 99 cent loaves of refined white sliced bread, $2 containers of milk and $3 bags of lollies. We hunt our food in convenient colourful packages, place them into wire cages and occasionally fight our neighbouring tribe for toilet paper. The padlock stays firmly on the storage shed.

Did you know that *every* fat cell we have, already exists in our body by the age of two? Those damn fat cells grow in size at almost unlimited capacity, like being able to put a new extension on the firewood shed.

Let's look at how our bodies fill up those fat cells.

Blood vessels are like superhighways—busy mass transit systems. Fat combos, called triglycerides, ride those highways. A triglyceride is made up of glycerol, a form of sugar, plus fatty acids. After it rides the freeway to the door of your fat cell, it can't enter by itself. It needs... drumroll please... insulin! Using an enzyme called lipoprotein lipase (LPL) that is stimulated by insulin, the triglyceride is chopped up into individual components to be stashed in the cell for storage. Without insulin to activate this enzyme, the components can't be stored.

Insulin opens the door, and once inside the cell, it's all reassembled and turned into a complete *storage form of fat*. To leave the fat cell and be used as energy, the triglyceride needs to be pulled apart by an enzyme called HSL (hormone-sensitive lipase) and, to add insult to injury, *high insulin levels turn off HSL.*

In other words, insulin blocks your fat from leaving the fat cell. Insulin is biochemically the cause of both weight gain and fat storage.

When insulin is high, the exit door remains locked and the fat can't leave. It's the guard at the castle door. Nobody in, nobody out. Your body can no longer access the essential stores of energy, and it creates hunger signals. At this point, *dammit*, you'll forage and devour that chocolate bar berating yourself later because you caved in, causing cortisol (another fat storage hormone) to spike. Your body is starving, and even though it has fat to burn, it can't access it, because insulin is on guard at the door.

Bear with me, we are nearly there...

If your insulin level remains too high (too many guards), for too long, a condition called *insulin resistance* occurs. Insulin resistance is created when your cells don't respond well anymore to insulin and you have lowered your ability to use glucose for energy, therefore you are *hungry*. And you hunt. Your willpower dissolves faster than you can say 'Mary Poppins'. In response, your pancreas produces *more* insulin to clear the sugar that is having a party in your blood like an uninvited house guest, trashing your system, leaving graffiti on the walls, and doing mass internal damage. This is known as type 2 diabetes.

Insulin resistance also occurs in the brain and has been labelled by scientists as type 3 diabetes. These locked brain cells are hungry. A hungry cell is a starving cell—starving cells die. Too much insulin for prolonged periods of time, a closed and guarded door, signals your body to eat quick energy foods. So, your willpower collapses. *Again.* Almost like being on autopilot, you are driven to give your hungry cells the fastest energy source you can get your hands on— this might be potato chips, a donut, chocolate or a bag of jelly snakes.

Our 'lack of willpower' is blamed but know that *it's not your fault*. Your body is driving you to this—Survival mode *on*.

Insulin resistance occurs over time—over 10, 20 or more years. As, gradually, our cells become more and more resistant to insulin, it often goes unnoticed. Diabetes is generally not diagnosed until the pancreas is exhausted and insulin levels are no longer enough to clear the excess blood sugar. Don't despair! You can reverse your diabetes and insulin resistance in a few short months.

This also explains why, as we age, it becomes increasingly difficult to burn our body fat, and why some of us gradually stack on the sizes. This also tends to be why it escapes our notice until it's too late, but if you're having issues with food cravings and willpower, it's worth considering the possibility you're becoming insulin resistant. You can be tested for this by asking your doctors to measure your insulin resistance through a test called HOMA-IR. Most of them aren't aware of this test—so persevere. Dr Eric Berg has a great video on this.

Alternatively, you can do some simple things to immediately lower your insulin response for some pretty fast results, as I have described in further chapters.

7 signs you may have insulin resistance:

- skin tags
- belly fat
- hungry all the time and at the mercy of cravings
- tired after a meal
- high blood pressure
- velvety patches of skin pigmentation
- tingling in your hands or feet

The brain on ketones

Those moments you walk into a room and forget why you are there—the ones we put down to 'senior moments'—aren't actually senior moments. They are caused, in part, by the deterioration in our brain, accelerated by insulin resistance.

Over time (decades) our brain loses the ability to effectively use glucose. Insulin resistance in the brain is a key factor linked to age-based cognitive impairment, for instance, ageing and memory loss. Recent evidence suggests that around the age of 47, our brain networks begin to destabilise, dramatically changing and deteriorating—and even more so, from the ages 60 and up.

Traditionally, glucose has been considered to be the brain's preferred fuel, however ketone metabolism has recently been proven to increase brain energy access by almost 30 per cent compared to glucose. Access to ketones also shows an increase in overall brain activity and better stabilised brain function[4]. Ketones, whether exogenous (taken in a drink) or endogenous (internally produced), bypass the guard at the door. This is referred to as the 'blood brain barrier'.

Ex-chairman of NASA, and keen brain researcher, Dr Ken Ford said: *'The brain is a greedy consumer of fuel, so it doesn't take much deprivation to observe change. Ketones improve cognitive performance and brain function, and communication between brain regions become more stable.'*

The vitally important role of ketones in the human brain starts in the womb and as a baby, you were born in a mild state of ketosis. Ketones are an essential fuel for a baby's brain because there is insufficient glucose available for energy requirements. This is thanks mostly to the fats present in breast milk. Human babies use this not only to build their brains, but to host significant fat stores, which any parent will attest to. Sweet, cuddly babies with their energy reserves in chubby rolls, ready for the time they crawl.

The adult brain is only about 2 per cent of our body weight, but this hungry control centre consumes 20–25 per cent of our energy intake. Because of this, the brain is particularly susceptible to metabolic changes. Like the rest of our body, the brain uses ketones for when glucose supply is disrupted, such as in times of starvation, long winters, fasting or prolonged exercise. Ketones are the *only significant alternative fuel source* to glucose for our brains and it's been proven that the brain prefers to run on ketones. Unlike glucose, ketones cross the blood brain barrier to our cells without the need for insulin, therefore providing these cells with an efficient fuel source, explaining the clarity of thought and improvement of mood many who follow a low carb lifestyle describe.

In a 2020 study, Dr Lilianne Mujica-Parodi, a thought leader in her field of brain research, proved that the brain will choose ketones preferentially over glucose, and that ketones can help reverse brain insulin resistance. Using new brain mapping technology, and large-scale life span data, this study showed that as we age, communication in the brain destabilises.

The study also showed that, while glucose *decreased* the stability of the brain networks, ketones *increased* it. Interestingly, this was observed across both adoption of a keto-style diet, as well as the use of natural bio-identical ketones.[1,2]

This study shows that, given the choice of the two fuels, our brains will choose to prioritise ketone bodies, whenever present. They are *immediately* used by the brain regardless, whereas glucose is only taken up by cells, as required. This study[5], saw stabilising effects on the brain, and explains why people describe clarity of thought and better mood, when they follow a keto or low-carb diet or consume a quality, naturally fermented bioidentical ketone. Ketones are not only a way of correcting fat storage issues, they also provide increased efficiency between networks in your brain.

'As we age, we can stabilise our neural pathways and lessen our chances of getting dementia and Alzheimer's by instead allowing ketones to fuel our brain.'
DR LILIANNE MUJICA-PARODI

Alzheimer's disease and diabetes are currently among the top threats to human health worldwide. A connection between these diseases has been established during the past decade, and an emerging body of evidence suggests that increased occurrence of *insulin resistance* contributes to Alzheimer's disease. The ketone molecule, regardless of whether it is endogenously made (in the body) or exogenously taken (into the body from an external source) has also been proven to show a positive effect on stabilising cognitive abilities in Alzheimer's diseased brains and those with mild cognitive impairment.

A Mayo Clinic study published in the *Journal of Alzheimer's Disease* found that those aged 70 and above with a higher-carbohydrate or high sugar diet, have over *three* times the risk of developing cognitive impairment, over those who followed low-carb or keto. The great news is that those whose lifestyles were highest in fat, were 42 per cent *less likely* to suffer from cognitive impairment than the participants whose diets were low in fat.

Research recently published in the New England Journal of Medicine shows that even slightly elevated levels of blood sugar (even too low to show risk of type 2 diabetes) still contributes to a significantly higher risk of developing dementia.

There are also many interesting, well documented studies around traumatic brain injuries and post traumatic disorders, studying the uptake of ketones vs. glucose in the brain, especially relating to neural regeneration, by researchers like Dr Stephen Cunane and Dr Stephen Phinney. You may also like to check *The Charlie Foundation* in regard to brain health and repairing cognitive function. Virtahealth.com also has real time statistics, particularly on reversing diabetes with nutrition.

Ketoacidosis vs. ketosis

No discussion on ketosis and its benefits would be complete without a quick word on ketoacidosis. Even though they sound the same, *ketosis and ketoacidosis are two very different things.*

Ketoacidosis refers todiabetic ketoacidosis, a complication of type 1 diabetes, which is a dangerous condition resulting in exceedingly high levels of ketones and blood sugar in the body (because of missing street sweepers). The blood becomes too acidic and changes the function of internal organs such as the liver and kidneys. There is almost *no* chance of this happening if you're following a keto or low-carb lifestyle, or if you are drinking natural, bio-identical ketones. If you're implementing this lifestyle as a type 1 diabetic, make sure you talk to your doctor so you can monitor your body changes.

Nutritional ketosis, in contrast, is a perfectly normal metabolic state where your body adapts to burning fat rather than carbohydrates or sugar as its primary fuel. Nutritional ketosis can be induced by following a ketogenic diet, where you lower carbs and increase healthy fats.

This all sounds great, Emma, but how do I follow and stick to a keto lifestyle when I crave the donuts?

You've heard it's hard. Actually, it isn't. It's just about consistently making sustainable, one step-at-a-time changes. Once you understand how to flip the metabolic switch, from burning the kindling all the time, minimising the guard at the door and not having to *constantly* replenish your energy, you'll be freed from the incessant craving rollercoaster.

I know this, because it happened to me. Instead, you can burn the logs in the shed. Because your body has access to both of its native fuel sources instead of just one and, even better, it understands how to use *both* of them, you can become metabolically flexible. Able to switch from one fuel source to the other, easily.

And that, is how we were meant to be.

Our genes have evolved over thousands of years to accommodate a high-fat, low-carb diet, however today we feed our bodies and brain almost the opposite.

It seems simple, doesn't it? Where did we go so very wrong?

CHAPTER 4

The big fat lie

> '*The most fattening foods are the ones that have the greatest effect on our blood sugar and insulin levels.*'
> GARY TAUBES, *WHY WE GET FAT AND WHAT TO DO ABOUT IT*

F at does not make us fat. This has been proven over and over. For some reason we still believe that fat is the enemy. Fat has been made into our Voldemort. We have been told (incorrectly) that fat in our diet is responsible for most of our current and ever-growing health afflictions. Search for the terms 'healthy fat' or 'keto' on the internet and suddenly, you're going to die a nasty, fat-clogged death. In actual fact, the very opposite is true. Fat is incredibly important, in fact, it's vital, and *absolutely essential* to our body and brain's basic functions.

The human brain is nearly 60 per cent fat.

All of our body parts depend on high-quality fat; however, the brain is uniquely vulnerable. Although your heart will also thank you for eating more fat, the brain is a direct beneficiary of omega-3 fats which are needed to spark communication between cells. Fat boosts cognition, happiness, learning and memory. Alternatively, a deficiency of omega-3 fatty acids has been linked to mood disorders like schizophrenia, depression, anxiety, bipolar disorders and even an increase in violent behaviour.

Fat is a macro nutrient, exactly like protein and carbohydrates. Your body *needs* fat for cushioning joints, building structure, and absorbing vitamins, plus protecting the health of your heart.

When we remove quality fats from our diet, we struggle with brain fog and clarity of thought, lack of satiety and experience issues with restorative sleep, mobility and cravings.

Brain foods high in omega-3 fatty acids

- fatty fish (salmon, mackerel, herring, sardines, anchovies)
- grass-fed animals
- dairy from grass-fed animals
- eggs from pastured chickens
- algae
- chia seeds, flaxseeds and hemp seeds
- walnuts
- avocados

Why do we believe fat is a killer?

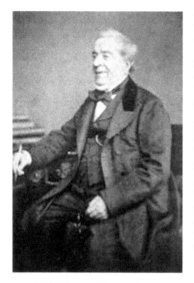

William Banting, one of the earliest successful adopters of a low carb lifestyle.

Banting was a portly English royal undertaker, who struggled, like many of us, with his girth well into his forties. Growing rounder, he sought assistance from doctors. One particular physician suggested that he 'eat less, move more', and so, on this suggestion, Banting rowed the river for a couple of hours every day, only to find that it served to intensify his hunger and prompted him to 'overindulge' afterwards.

Banting tried everything that was recommended, from bathing to ear burning, without seeing any positive change, and in frustration turned to his friend and physician, Dr William Harvey. With Dr Harvey's assistance, he made some dietary changes, such as limiting the intake of carbohydrates, 'especially those of a starchy or sugary nature', and quickly saw results like better sleep and mobility, improved eyesight, and of course—fat loss—to the tune of 38 pounds (17 kilograms) in 38 weeks. He was excited, as he considered this diet to be a 'generous and extravagant one'.

He got so passionate about this discovery, it led him to penning a personal testimonial in 1863 called *Letter on Corpulence, addressed to the Public*, in which he spoke of his previously unsuccessful diets and exercise regimes, prescribed by various doctors and his excitement about finding something that worked.

'Said my excellent adviser, starch and saccharine matter, tending to create fat, should be avoided altogether' he wrote. 'Within a very few days, I found immense benefit from it.'

Banting continued, *'My girth is reduced round the waist, in tailor phraseology, twelve-and-a-quarter inches, which extent was hardly conceivable even by my own friends, or my respected medical adviser, until I put on my former clothing, over what I now wear, which was a thoroughly convincing proof of the remarkable change.'*

Banting and Harvey are credited for being among the first to popularise low-carb weight loss. 'To bant' is a term used to this day referring to a low carb lifestyle.

He wasn't alone in his discovery. In the early 1920s, University of Michigan physician, Dr Louis Newburgh, documented his successful treatment of diabetics using *only* nutrition. He published many articles on the remarkable effectiveness of low-carb diets while treating his patients. Dr Newburgh said, *'Every attempt was made to avoid all carbohydrate.'*

Even in the household, early post-war food ration articles advised 'cutting down on bread, potatoes and carrots for losing weight'. A *Woman's Own* magazine article from 1945 suggested women exercise caution at mealtimes, since *'war-time rationing has led to an increased consumption of starchy fattening foods, with unflattering results to our figures.'* The article recommended that, in order to lose fat, the women should reduce the number of meals and cut down on bread, potato, cakes and biscuits.

This message was repeated many times in *Woman's Own magazine* throughout the years. Following this simple plan, they said, would *'tackle those surplus pounds amassed during winter, a season which,' according to Woman's Own, 'has a nasty habit of adding curves we don't need'.*

In the early 1950s, George Cahill, a former professor of medicine at Harvard Medical School pioneered information on human metabolism and blood glucose. He stated that *'carbohydrate is driving insulin is driving fat,'* and went on to research many breakthroughs in diabetes reversal using ketosis and nutrition.

By the mid-1950s, some of the brightest doctors in the world, from renowned universities like Harvard, Stanford and Columbia, were publishing articles advocating for lower-carb diets to treat obesity and diabetes. They shared the advice for their patients to eat as much red meat, fish, chicken, eggs, fats, cheese and green vegetables as they liked, while avoiding carbohydrate-rich foods and drinks, particularly sweets.

Also, in the 1950s, Dr Benjamin Spock (I just love his name—it speaks to my inner Star Trekkie) taught the same principle, in the *Bible of Child-Rearing* saying, *'Rich desserts and the amount of plain, starchy foods (cereals, breads, potatoes) taken, is what determines, in the case of most people, how much [weight] they gain or lose.'*

By the end of the 1950s, fears of a growing coronary heart epidemic led a frantic search for the culprit.

In 1955, American President Eisenhower suffered a heart attack. He made details of his illness public. His chief physician, Dr Paul Dudley White, held a press conference the following day, where he gave Americans instruction on how to avoid the dreaded heart disease. His suggestions: stop smoking, cut saturated fat and therefore minimise cholesterol. He cited work by the American nutritionist, Ancel Keys, and research from the University of Minnesota.

During this time, nutritionists and scientists split into two distinct groups. One group followed Ancel Keys and believed wholeheartedly that dietary fat was to blame for the rising epidemic. On the opposing side, among others, were statisticians, Jacob Yerushalmy and Herman Hilleboe and English nutritionist, Dr John Yudkin, who believed that it wasn't fat, but sugar that was responsible.

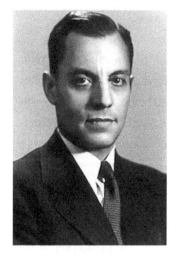

Dr Ancel Keys was born in 1904 in Colorado Springs, USA. An oceanographer, turned physiologist, he was intelligent, blunt and extremely persuasive.

In 1958, Keys launched a major survey regarding the risk of cardiovascular disease. The conclusion of this study stated that an excess of saturated fats from our traditional fare—red meat, cheese, butter and eggs was responsible for raised cholesterol, therefore leading to coronary disease. He recommended that following a diet low in fat would therefore reduce cholesterol. He blamed fat for clogging arteries causing them to harden and narrow, restricting the flow of blood to the heart. However, there was *no credible evidence* to support this theory.

You can see, in retrospect, why this makes sense. In our mind's eye, we can paint a picture of that bacon fat or butter sitting in a clump in our blood vessels. Unfortunately, even though incorrect, this image made people very scared of dietary fat.

Senator George McGovern implemented the guidelines suggested by Keys almost immediately. He and the nutritional elite boys club, most of whom knew or worked with each other, all agreed that fat was the problem.

McGovern, Eisenhower, Keys and Dudley-White were a united, powerful megaphone, and the notion that fat was unhealthy started to take hold, especially with doctors, who wanted to help their patients. Eisenhower too, it's worth noting, amended his diet to follow the advice and proceeded to *exclude* saturated fats from his diet until his death in 1969 when he passed away from... can you guess?

Heart disease, despite having adopted a low-fat diet.

The slimming advice had changed. We were now encouraged to prepare more elaborate meals, lower our fat, increase carbohydrate intake and significantly limit portion sizes and count calorie content. Due to consumer demand, food manufacturers started to lower the fat content in their products on the basis that it was supposedly killing us. They had to add the flavour back in somehow though, because fat makes things taste great. When they took fat out, they added... drumroll, please... you guessed it!

Sugar.

Seven Countries Study

The Seven Countries Study was the first major study to investigate diet and lifestyle over an extended period of time, looking for risk factors for cardiovascular disease across contrasting cultures and countries. The countries were chosen for lifestyle, eating habits and risk factor levels. The study included 22 countries; however, Keys chose to publish and correlate *just 7*, in support of his hypothesis, that fat was the cause of heart disease.

Even at this point, a growing number of researchers and scientists disagreed vehemently with Keys' analysis. Many believed that his concept lacked any solid evidence, and in fact, that his proof was simplistic, but he was convinced he was correct. There was no basis for his country selection—only those countries that supported his beliefs were chosen for the conclusion. As an example, he left out France and Germany who had fairly low heart disease rates, despite living on a happy diet rich in saturated fats.

The Seven Countries Study had two other major issues. Firstly, it was a correlation study that didn't prove causation, making it easy to jump to incorrect conclusions. The other issue was that to reliably identify *cause*, a higher standard of evidence would have been required, such as a randomised controlled trial. This is a study where researchers recruit a group, assign half of the participants a particular diet for a certain period of time, and the other half another—then at the end, assessing those in each group vs. the other, but this wasn't the case.

Many years later, Alessandro Menotti, the study's lead researcher, re-reviewed the data and found the food that linked more closely with deaths, was not saturated fat but, in fact, *sugar*.

The study was also disproven by two statisticians, Yerushalmy and Hilleboe, who created their own graph from the full 22 countries, and showed a weakened correlation between total fat and heart disease, rather than the definitive proof Keys had offered. There were also many studies, including the Women's Health Initiative (some 30 years later) that disproved Keys' theories!

By that time, the belief was like a freight train, powering towards its destination—*unstoppable*. The low-fat, calorie-counting movement had gained so much momentum that it carries on to this day, despite large bodies of evidence that directly contradict this theory.

Cholesterol

Cholesterol was also standing at the bus stop right beside fat when the car crashed into it. It isn't the health villain either, that it's been made out to be—in fact, it's *so* important, we can't live without it. There are several kinds of cholesterol our bodies make and it's important they aren't all lumped in together, because some cholesterol is essential.

This cholesterol is *so vitally important* that our *own* liver makes it and if we don't have enough, we make more. It's required as a conductor for chemical messages between neurons and is the building block of every cell membrane. It's used in the same way as essential fats, to create new cells including those responsible for memory and cognition.

It's also used for key hormone production such as testosterone and estrogen. Cholesterol helps produce bile, needed to digest and absorb fats, and its role in processing vitamin D is of vital importance. It's also absolutely necessary for the health of our immune system.

An opposing viewpoint of Keys' diet-heart hypothesis was held by Dr. John Yudkin, who found in his studies, that sugar correlated with heart disease perfectly. He put forward an opposing view that high sugar consumption was a key cause of heart disease. This was met with *massive* vocal opposition from Keys and his colleagues.

Dr John Yudkin was born in the East End, London, in 1910. He was qualified in biochemistry and physiology before becoming interested in nutrition science medicine. He was struck by the data

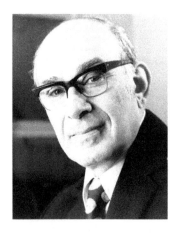

he was seeing on high consumption of sugar rather than fat and he focussed his efforts on the study of sugar and its effect on the body. He observed that sugar turned to fat in the liver.

In his 1972 book, *Pure, White and Deadly*, Yudkin states that everything from diabetes to obesity, from hyperactivity to eczema and arthritis, can all be traced back to sugar.

Yudkin wrote:

'If only a small fraction of what we know about the effects of sugar were to be revealed in relation to any other material used as a food additive, that material would promptly be banned.'

His book did exceptionally well, but he paid dearly for it.

The war was on.

At the time the Seven Countries Study was published, Yudkin wrote to *The Lancet*, a well-respected science journal, to accuse Keys of presenting *'awkward facts'* and *'cherry-picking only the data which supported their view'*.

Keys publicly ridiculed Yudkin and accused him of propaganda for the meat and dairy industries in an attempt to discredit him. Yudkin never responded, however, it made him highly vulnerable to attack. Keys had accumulated some *very* powerful friends and had secured elevated places on boards in American healthcare institutions. Needless to say, Keys' unproven theory about fat being Voldemort won.

70

The Framingham Study

From 1948, the University of Harvard ran a 12 year long, community-wide study of habits in a town called Framingham, Massachusetts. Even today, it is one of the world's longest running nutrition studies. Every few years, residents of this whole town completed blood tests and polls. The researchers were hoping to find a definitive link between saturated dietary fat, blood cholesterol and heart disease, however, instead they found...

Nothing at all.

There was absolutely *no proof* over those 12 years, that dietary fat was *in any way* responsible for the growing epidemic of heart disease. The findings were *actually* that saturated fats were *not* responsible for increased blood cholesterol.

'No association between per cent of calories from fat and serum cholesterol level was shown; nor between ratio of plant fat to animal fat intake and serum cholesterol level... There is, in short, no suggestion of any relation between diet and the subsequent development of CHD [coronary heart disease] in the study group.'

Dr Ancel Keys was also the lead investigator in the 1968 study, the Minnesota Coronary Experiment, that took place in a nursing home and six state mental hospitals over five years, involving almost 10,000 subjects. This study replaced saturated fat with omega-6 fatty acids (vegetable oils) and found that it did in fact reduce cholesterol. However, shockingly, the *more cholesterol measurements fell, the greater the mortality* rate. This information was never published and it wasn't until 2016 that the information was extracted from dusty vaults and the findings published in the British Medical Journal.

'Available evidence from randomised controlled trials shows that replacement of saturated fat in the diet with linoleic acid effectively lowers serum cholesterol but does not support the hypothesis that this translates to a lower risk of death from coronary heart disease or all causes.'

Over the next 50 years, history repeated. No matter how intently researchers peered into the correlations, there was absolutely *no* direct relationship between dietary fat and blood cholesterol.

When you are warned about high fat intake and you're told your cholesterol will increase, know that the truth is, in fact, the very opposite of what many believe, and is a *myth* that has been disproven over and over again.

The Puerto Rico Heart Health Program—this program was a huge study with over 10,000 patients. The results were the same. Heart disease could not be linked to dietary fat.

Nurses' Health Study—this study followed over 80,000 nurses for 14 years and concluded that *'total fat intake is not significantly related to the risk of coronary disease.'* Dietary cholesterol was also deemed safe.

Siri-Tarino PW meta-analysis—an analysis by Dr R Krause of 21 studies involving over 340,000 patients found *'no significant evidence for dietary saturated fat being associated with increased risk of chronic heart disease.'*

Today, many highly credible researchers and passionate foodies champion this conversation, including: Jamie Oliver; Dr Tim Noakes, Dr Gary Fettke, Dr Paul Mason, a young, intelligent and promising Australian doctor; Dr Jason Fung, who is successfully reversing patients diabetes in Canada using intermittent fasting and low-carb nutrition; Dr Robert Lustig, the next generation of anti-sugar campaigners; Gary Taubes, researcher and outspoken journalist, who combs the PubMed journals; and Nina Teicholz, who is smart, funny and incredibly gifted at explaining the yawning holes in knowledge. And my own local doctor—a young and passionate champion of the nutrition conversation. These and many, many others have broken apart and highlighted the flaws in this incorrect diet hypothesis.

Let thy food be thy medicine and medicine be thy food

You've heard this phrase before. Nutrition has been a central element in many traditional cultures until its role declined, with the increasing amounts of medications prescribed during the last century, curing almost every ailment we suffer from. The issue is that these medications generally treat the symptom, not the cause. Recently, increased awareness of the importance of lifestyle and nutrition for disease prevention has signalled winds of change, and a U-turn in beliefs about food as nutrition.

Let thy food be thy medicine... when possible

There is now (and always has been) a large body of evidence suggesting that nutrition can reduce disease and treat the cause of many ailments we currently treat with medications. General lifestyle interventions as opposed to prescriptions for health and well-being, are being explored alongside nutritional strategies to stabilise or even reverse diseases directly associated with a high blood sugar lifestyle. Some of these diseases are obesity, cardio-vascular disease, type 2 diabetes, polycystic ovarian syndrome (PCOS), depression, bowel diseases, Parkinson's disease, fibromyalgia, MS, IBS, Alzheimer's and dementia.

So, just in case I've freaked you out and you don't make it any further in this book, here are some little changes you can implement straight away.

Small changes for a super-powered brain:

- Don't drink your sugar.
- Be aware of what spikes your blood sugar—therefore raises insulin levels (even if you're not diabetic).
- Understand that *insulin is a fat storage hormone* (yes, I said it again).
- Invest in a blood glucose/ketone monitor—knowing what spikes your blood sugar (read: fat storage) is key.
- Eat healthy fats. Fat improves satiety, and in turn, offers better control over impulse food choices.
- Eat a rainbow of *seasonal* vegetables.
- Check the back of your labels and choose *no added sugar*.
- Give up the junk. You'll save you money too.
- Cook at home using healthy fats like butter, ghee and coconut or olive oil.
- Toss the processed seed oils.
- Google keto and low carb versions of your favourite foods.
- If you can't pronounce the ingredient, *don't buy it*.
- Shop the outside of the aisles. Start with fresh, real food.

CHAPTER 5

What the fat?

A dding healthy fat to your diet helps you feel satisfied after a meal, reducing hunger and therefore promoting weight loss. Fat activates the satiety hormone, leptin, which means fewer cravings, less pantry door-swinging, and banishing late-night snack attacks.

Healthy fats help us to:

- absorb more nutrients
- increase 'good' HDL cholesterol and lower damaging LDL cholesterol
- lower the risk of stroke and heart disease
- fight inflammation
- lower blood pressure
- improve hormone function
- improve memory

- improve joint mobility
- prevent early onset of dementia and Alzheimer's
- prevent atherosclerosis (hardening and narrowing of the arteries)
- improve cognition

It's not eating fat that makes you store fat. It's eating the *wrong* types of fat.

Oils ain't oils

Tossing the majority of vegetable oils straight into the bin is one of the simplest steps you can take for your family's health. A relatively new introduction to our lives, many of todays processed foods include cheap, poor-quality fats (omega-6) from refined vegetable oils, and the bulk of them host sugar in some form as well. It's the combination of these two ingredients that is *particularly* damaging, leading to systematic inflammation. (Read as—the donut, the fries, the snack foods).

Vegetable oils on supermarket shelves today, were developed at the end of the 19th century, when technological advances allowed oils to be extracted from plant crops. Even a hundred years ago, there were very few vegetable oils in our food—these did not form a significant part of our diet at all.

With the overzealous adoption of the low-fat movement, we were advised to ditch our traditional fats, that human-beings have consumed for tens of thousands of years and embrace seed oils instead. Today's mass-produced vegetable oils require *significant* industrial processing using emulsifiers and other chemical techniques to combine water and chemically refined vegetable oils, creating shelf stability, however at the same time, unfortunately damaging our gut health. Sunflower, linseed, palm and canola, with added preservatives, flavourings and vitamins are combined, using processes such as heat, cold, high-speed spinning, solvents like hexane, degumming agents, deodorisers and bleaching agents, to process seeds into a palatable, food-friendly long-lasting oil.

Did you know that in 1869, oleomargarine (later shortened to 'margarine') was patented and invented by French Chemist, Hippolyte Mège-Mouriès, in response to a challenge by Emperor Napoleon III. A prize was offered to anyone who could produce a cheap butter alternative for use in his army and to provide for the lower classes. Originally it was a combination of beef fat and skim milk (butter removed). Dutch company Jurgens purchased the patent (which later became part of Unilever) and still makes Flora margarine today, but this was a much healthier option than what was to follow.

For the first time in 1871, Henry W. Bradley patented the process that made margarine spreadable—a highly desirable trait—it was made using cottonseed oil combined with animal fats. The early 20th century also saw the invention of chemical processes that turned vegetable oils into solid fats, known as hydrogenation.

The revolution of vegetable oils began.

After the First World War, the Great Depression of the 1930s led to a mass shortage of animal fats, which in turn created the perfect environment for the margarine industry to grow their reputation as a budget-friendly alternative to butter. Food shortages were common and pre-packaged food was on the rise, not only for armed troops, but for most of the European population. Food needed to be transported across great distances to those in need without spoiling.

The invention of long-lasting hydrogenated vegetable oils opened the door for Big Food to find its way into every household. Terrific marketing campaigns ensured that, in a very short space of time, by targeting housewives with cookbooks and the like, these damaging oils became integrated into every single kitchen pantry.

In the 1970s, supported by international medical societies, campaigns against saturated fats used Keys' hypothesis for great market advantage leading to a perfect storm—these oils had become fashionable and were marketed as the 'right choice'. In response to high consumer demand, fast-food companies switched from traditional fats, to hydrogenated oils containing trans-fats.

Hydrogenation chemically alters vegetable oils in the manufacturing process to ensure they stay solid at room temperature—it gives them a longer shelf life. Hydrogenation also increases flavour and stability and can be spotted in an impressive list of foods including vegetable oils, margarine, crackers (even healthy sounding ones), cereals, lollies, baked goods, biscuits, granola bars, chips, snack foods, salad dressings, fats, fried foods, and many other processed foods in your own pantry. Your favourite restaurant probably uses partially hydrogenated vegetable oil in their deep fryer, so they don't have to change the oil as often.

These oils, although appealing to Big Food, because of cost and transportability, are, unfortunately not a great choice for our health.

Recent medical research has revealed serious health implications regarding most of these oils—as they are reheated repeatedly to high temperatures, they develop toxic, carcinogenic elements.

Consumption of only five grams of these oils per day is associated with a *23 per cent increase* in the risk of coronary heart disease. These processed oils promote inflammation, as does sugar, and the combination that we love so much (donuts) leads to a ticking time bomb inside our body. This combo causes massive, systemic inflammation. Inflammation is at the root of nearly every chronic disease, especially those impacting the brain and the heart.

Processed oils have also been linked to risk of multiple diseases including cardiovascular disease and cancer. Trans-fats increase the risk of developing type 2 diabetes, stroke, insulin resistance and triglycerides—while at the same time lowering healthy cholesterol that is imperative for cell repair and brain function.

Ahead of the game, Denmark was the first to place a ban on the sale of products containing trans-fats in 2003. Austria, Hungary, Iceland, Norway and Switzerland have now set similar limits that ban trans-fats from use in food products.

We were told that vegetable oils were good, and butter was bad. We were told that traditional fats (like our grandparents ate, and their parents before them), like tallow, ghee, lard, butter and coconut oil caused high cholesterol and clogged our arteries, leading to heart disease. Blaming cholesterol for heart disease is like blaming a fire fighter for starting the fire, instead of being at the scene to resolve the issue. Cholesterol is the fixit of our bodies, and often seen at the sight of inflammation and doing its job of repair—not causing it, as widely believed.

There is no doubt that the practices of replacing saturated fats with trans-fat products, in conjunction with the dietary guidelines of 1978 have resulted in an increase of cardiovascular diseases.

Exactly what they were trying to avoid.

What you can do

- Toss out omega-6-rich, inflammatory polyunsaturated fats.
- Check out the ingredients on your packets: if the list includes oils like corn, soy, cottonseed or safflower, you'd be better to leave it on the supermarket shelf.

Industrial seed oils to *avoid* include canola, corn, cottonseed soy, sunflower, safflower, grapeseed, rice bran and margarine.

Healthy fats to *include* in your diet include coconut oil, avocado oil, lard (pork fat), tallow (rendered beef or mutton fat), butter, ghee, olive oil and MCT oil.

Choose:

- fattier cuts of meat—often cheaper too!
- avocados—natures perfect package of fibre and fat.
- ghee, lard and coconut oil—these are the best cooking fats.
- olive oil—look for dark glass that prevents oxidisation and dose liberally on your salads.
- MCT oil—helps your brain function and regenerate neural pathways and also helps your liver make its own ketones.
- butter—self-explanatory and yum!
- olives—preferably not in canola oil.
- fatty fish—fresh (not canned) tuna, herrings, mackerel,

salmon, sardines and trout. If choosing canned, buy marinated in brine or olive oil, not canola.

- dark chocolate—choose over 80 per cent cocoa solids and look for low sugar content. It's rich in magnesium, potassium and calcium. Have a square to help kill the late-night cravings.
- eggs—natures perfect oval combo of fat and protein.
- nuts—brazil, walnuts, pecans, macadamias and almonds are especially good—make sure to eat in moderation if fat loss is a goal for you.
- seeds—chia and flaxseeds—two of the best plant-based omega-3 sources you can get.

Signs you're not getting enough quality 'good' dietary fat:
- dry, flaking or itchy, skin
- cravings
- soft, brittle cracked nails
- aching joints
- tiny bumps on the backs of your arms or torso (did you just feel the back of your arm?)
- depression
- memory and cognition problems
- attention deficit disorder
- diabetes
- weight gain

A few friendly fat recipes

CHIA PUDDING (3 STEPS)

Ingredients
3 tbs chia seeds
1 cup sugar-free nut milk or coconut milk
Keto friendly sweetener (if required) such as erythritol or monkfruit—add to taste

Instructions
Stir together chia seeds and milk in a jar or bowl. For a thicker chia pudding, try 4 tbs chia seeds to 1 cup of liquid. Once well-combined, allow to sit for a few minutes, give it another stir to break up any clumps of the seeds, cover and put the mixture in the fridge to set for 1–2 hours or overnight. Add sweetener as desired.

The chia pudding should be nice and thick. If it's not thick, just add more chia seeds (1 tsp to 1 tbs), stir and refrigerate for another 30 minutes or so. To this, you can add a few berries or some sugar-free maple syrup, sweetener or MCT oil if desired.

See the chapter on sugar and alternatives for other options.

A dairy-free twist for chocolate lovers:
Combine 1 ½ tbs chia seeds,1 tbs cacao, 1 tsp powdered erythritol, ½ cup unsweetened nut milk, ¼ cup coconut cream. Follow the above process.

EASY KETO LEMON CURD

Ingredients
4 egg yolks
¼ cup erythritol or monkfruit
25 grams butter
2 large lemons, zested and juiced

Instructions
In a small saucepan, on low heat, whisk the egg yolks and erythritol together.

Whisk until erythritol has dissolved.

Add the butter and lemon zest and continue whisking until the butter is melted. Lastly, add the lemon juice and continue whisking over medium heat until thickened.

Transfer to sterile jars or small ramekins and refrigerate until set.

BREAKFAST EGG MUFFINS

Filing and family friendly

Ingredients
10 large eggs
1–1 ½ tsp sea salt to taste
¼ - ½ tsp black pepper to taste
½ tsp dried thyme
½ tsp garlic powder
1 ½ cups broccoli, steamed and chopped (or frozen and thawed)
⅔ cup grated cheddar cheese, plus more for topping

Method
Preheat oven to 200°C. Grease a muffin tray with non-stick cooking spray. Set aside.

In a large mixing bowl, whisk eggs, salt and pepper.

Whisk in garlic powder and thyme until combined. Stir in broccoli and cheese. Divide evenly across a muffin tray so each hole is about two-thirds full.

Sprinkle with more cheddar if desired. Bake in preheated oven for 12–15 minutes or until set.

KETO SEED CRACKERS

Ingredients
⅓ cup almond flour
⅓ cup sunflower seeds
⅓ cup pumpkin seeds
⅓ cup flaxseed or chia seeds
⅓ cup sesame seeds
1 tbs psyllium husk powder
1 tsp pink salt
¼ cup melted coconut oil
1 cup boiling water

Method
Preheat the oven to 150°C. Mix all dry ingredients in a bowl. Add boiling water and oil. Mix together and keep working the dough until it forms a ball and has a gel-like consistency. Place the dough on a silicone mat or piece of quality baking paper. Add another piece of baking paper on top. Use a rolling pin to flatten the dough evenly and thinly. The thinner it is, the crispier it will be. Remove the upper paper and bake on the lower rack for about 40–45 minutes. Seeds are heat sensitive, so pay close attention towards the end.

Turn off oven and leave the crackers to dry *in the oven*. Once dried and cool, break into pieces and spread a generous amount of butter or avocado on top to consume.

CHAPTER 6

Voldemort

> 'Sugar's not dangerous because of its calories, or because it makes you fat. Sugar is dangerous because it's sugar. It's not nutrition. When consumed in excess, it's a toxin. And it's addictive.'
>
> ROBERT LUSTIG, MD,
> *THE TOXIC TRUTH ABOUT SUGAR*

Sugar has *always* called to me. My mum used to hide the lollies at various places in the top of the cupboard. Those golden jersey caramels in the glass recycled coffee jar called lovingly to me. I regularly scaled and scoured the pantry shelves looking for mum's next creative hiding place, after she'd found I'd raided the jar and she'd moved it to the next hiding spot. It became like a game of seek-and-reward for me. Hi Mum, if you're reading this, and sorry! I appreciate you!

The sugar 'hit' also led me to sneak out before primary school with my friends, down the road to the local juice factory, where we bought chocolate bars and lollies with our pocket money, and we stuffed our mouths as full as we could with the sweet delights before we were discovered. I paid for getting caught on that escapade with a leather belt across my bottom. Looking back, I guess my parents were worried about my safety instead of looking at *why* I was chasing the sugar. Sweet foods continuously called to me… this pattern repeated itself throughout my adulthood, when I'd hide coveted treats in the second drawer of my desk where nobody else could discover them, like a safety net of comfort.

Have you ever found yourself staring at the empty bag of biscuits you just inhaled in front of Netflix without knowing why? The family block of Cadbury Dairy Milk chocolate that you swore you'd only have a row of, that now lies demolished before you?

Don't beat yourself up. Remember, your brain is wired to look for sweet temptation—it's an automatic survival instinct.

Have you ever heard the term the 'bliss point'? It's a phrase coined by American market researcher and psychophysicist, Howard Moskowitz. The 'bliss point' is considered the perfect balance of ingredients, such as salt, sugar and fat, that optimises taste and food experience. A packet of Twisties or a delicious donut springs to mind. Food manufacturers spend *millions* creating that perfect, irresistible and addictive combo that makes us reach for more. It's the secret weapon manufacturers hold over us, in our world of packaged food today.

Unfortunately, sugar bypasses our normal fullness mechanisms, which is why you can stuff your face full of sweet treats all day, every day and not feel full. The more we do this, the less sensitive our body becomes to these foods, so you have to eat more to get the same rush. On the flip side, we experience withdrawal if we don't get it. It's like a readily available designer drug, in an easy-to-open resealable package any time we want it. How convenient.

> The global industrial sugar market is expected to reach US$45.6 billion by the year 2027. We love it and we crave it.

Sugar is also an important economic commodity. It's Australia's second largest crop for export after wheat and is worth annually almost AUD $2 billion. As you can imagine, the sugar associations of the world are not only powerful, but many livelihoods rely on this drug. It's big business.

The Australian sugar industry put publicly on the internet this statement:

*'At an average of 50 kilograms per capita per year, Australian sugar consumption exceeds that of European countries at around 40 kilograms per year, the United States of America at 33 kilograms and Japan at 20 kilograms. The Australian industry is constantly monitoring domestic sugar consumption and attitudes to sugar and adapts its marketing strategies and educational material as needed.'*12

What the. Just what the f... There's another F-word!

Fifty freaking kilograms per person, per year! That's almost a kilogram per week, per person. And did you miss the bit at the end where they are strategizing and marketing to us, so we consume even more?

Currently the WHO recommends a maximum of six teaspoons of sugar a day for females and slightly more for males—which incidentally is *six* times more than we are designed to have in our bloodstream. On average, Australians consume somewhere between

14–16 teaspoons of *added* sugar a day, and the figure is much higher in other parts of the world.

A 600 millilitre bottle of soft drink contains *16 teaspoons of sugar*. A bottle a day, is the equivalent of consuming 23 kilograms of sugar, just from soft drinks alone—*every* year. That's even before we take into account the sugar that is added into our food.

Easy sources of six teaspoons of sugar include:

- Large serve Nutri-Grain cereal (60 grams)
- Low-fat fruit yoghurt (200 grams)
- Glass of Coke (240 millilitres)
- Can of Red Bull (250 millilitres)
- Two-thirds of a bottle of Gatorade (400 millilitres)
- BBQ sauce (50 millilitres)
- ¾ Glass of Orange juice (250 millilitres)

Sugar is, at the same time, known to be the leading cause of obesity and disease worldwide. Medical professionals and epidemiologists all maintain that sugar consumption *directly* corresponds with chronic disease.

Sugar suppresses your immune system. It increases stress, cortisol levels and leads to fat storage. Sugar accelerates ageing through a process called glycation. Sugar causes tooth decay and leads to gum disease. Sugar affects behaviour and cognition in children (as all parents know). Sugar causes inflammation and creates massive insulin spikes, leading to insulin resistance. To add insult to injury—a high-sugar diet often results in chromium deficiency, one of the minerals that helps us regulate our blood sugar.

Studies on sugar consumption, show increased risk of chronic disease including obesity, cardiovascular disease, diabetes and non-alcoholic fatty liver disease as well as cognitive decline and even some cancers. Sugar feeds abnormal cell growth (think tumours and cancer). A fabulous TED talk to watch regarding this is *Starving Cancer* by Dr Dominic D'Agostino.

Sugar is addictive

Have you ever been on the sugar rollercoaster? I'm sure you have. I didn't even know I was on it. I was being *called* by the donuts. Seriously, I swear I could hear them calling to me from the other end of the shopping centre.

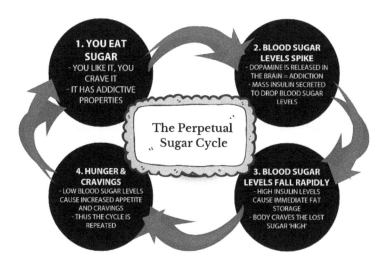

Sugar works on the reward and craving loop in the brain. It's actually more rewarding than cocaine and it's definitely more readily available, behaving like a drug in our bodies. In animal studies, sugar has been found to produce enough symptoms to be considered an addictive substance. In both animals and humans, evidence shows parallels between abused drugs and sugar. In its 'pure' white crystalline form, it is highly absorbable directly into our bloodstream. This leads to massive insulin spikes and release of dopamine (the happy hormone), causing us to want more, and making it very difficult to say no to.

Data has shown sugar's significant drug-like effects on brain neurochemistry as well as altered behaviour, including bingeing, cravings, tolerance, and withdrawal. It alters our mood, willpower and induces powerful cravings like an opioid.

In other words, it's habit-forming—just like cocaine, heroin, alcohol, tobacco, nicotine, tea, sex, coffee and chocolate. Don't get me wrong—keep the chocolate, let's just make a better chocolate choice (over 80 per cent cocoa solids). Let's keep the coffee too, of course. Just with no sugar, using non-spiking sugar replacements.

Addiction is a physiological dependence. After several weeks or months of chronic sugar intake, if you then decrease sugar levels it can lead to dopamine deficiency in the brain, caused by a reduction in our 'feel good' receptors. When dopamine levels drop, withdrawal occurs. We want more.

Obesity, ADHD and drug addiction all share the same trigger of downregulation of dopamine D2 receptors in the brain with symptoms such as hyperactivity, attention-deficit, distraction and decreased performance.

Sugar and refined carbohydrates (which have the same effect on our bodies as sugar) also have an effect on serotonin levels. After consuming a high-sugar meal, there is a spike in serotonin. Serotonin is the hormone that is responsible for stabilising our mood, and feelings of well-being and happiness, and you'll recognise it as the 'sleep' hormone.

Welcome to an endless cycle of highs and lows, sugar intake and dependence. Sugar (and other carbs such as complex sugars) make us feel better. Simple.

I hope you get a sense of the magnitude of what you're dealing with, and why the struggles you're facing aren't your fault. We are products of our 'easy food' environment.

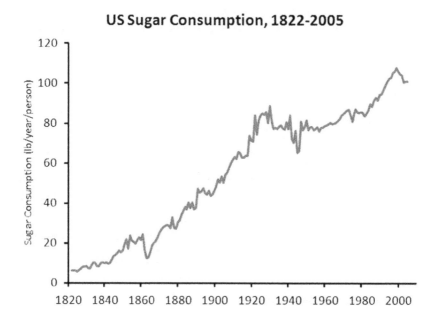

Sugar consumption is on the rise.

I went to school in Nambour on Queensland's Sunshine Coast—smack bang in the middle of one of Australia's most lush and productive sugarcane areas. The cane trains clattered through the middle of town with their big wire cages full of cut cane ready for the mill. In summer harvest season, black ash from burning cane in preparation for harvest would land all over our schoolbooks. During school excursions, we visited this local mill many times and were educated on the sugar processes. Even as a child, I remember being amazed by the number of processes and treatments sugar undergoes to land on our tables.

Historically, sugarcane first appeared on the tropical Pacific Islands of New Guinea 10,000 years ago, then made its way to India, crept east towards China and travelled with the trade routes to Persia as a valuable commodity. From the Islamic states, sugar meandered its way to Europe via the Crusaders, who brought back sugar from their journeys in the Holy Land. These travellers had encountered caravans carrying 'sweet salt'.

The first record of sugar in England is in the late 13th century. At this time, cane sugar remained an expensive resource and was mainly afforded by royalty—it was so precious, it was locked in boxes so the house staff couldn't sneak it. Its price per pound in medieval England was as high as imported spices from Asia, such as nutmeg, ginger, cloves and pepper, which were transported and traded across the Indian Ocean. When Christopher Columbus made his second voyage across the Atlantic Ocean in 1493, he brought with him sugar cane stalks as precious cargo. Sugar spread to the West Indies and was cultivated in the warmer regions in America, beginning in the 16th century.

Sugar was traditionally locally consumed and was little more than an exotic spice, however it was incredibly labour intensive. It had a very high value and, once refined, could be traded and transported over long distances by ship at a generous profit. The European sugar era began with the shift of production to Cyprus. They struggled to get local labourers for the taxing and dangerous work in the cane fields, so they brought in slaves from the Black Sea and Africa. It was the introduction of sugar slavery that made sugar affordable.

> *'The true Age of Sugar had begun—and it was doing more to reshape the world than any ruler, empire or war had ever done.'*
> MARC ARONSON AND MARINA BUDHOS,
> *SUGAR CHANGED THE WORLD*

Over the next 400 years, almost 11 million Africans were enslaved. Fuelled by the wealth of Europe, 'white gold' boomed. People were traded, profits were made. As Europeans established mass sugar plantations on the larger Caribbean islands, prices fell in Europe. By the 18th century, all levels of society had become common consumers of the formerly luxury product, through to today where it is readily available in all forms, directly from our supermarket shelves.

Sugar is in *so* many of our foods. The majority of sugar can be found in the bottled drinks aisle and in the baking aisle at the supermarket. Yet more is found in confectionery, bakery items, preserved foods, the bottle shop and dairy products.

One of the simplest changes towards 'better' you can make, is to check your packaging for *hidden* sugars.

Over the last 70 years, there have been some very vocal anti-sugar campaigners, including Dr John Yudkin, who we heard about last chapter. Professor Robert H. Lustig, an American paediatric endocrinologist believes that food business and the sugar industry have hacked our bodies and minds by way of addiction. He states that, *'focusing on real food you can beat the odds—against sugar, processed food, obesity and disease,'* and I'm inclined to agree, having been one of the people who has fortunately managed to break the addiction.

That Sugar Film released in 2014 reality-slapped me in the face. Director Damon Gameau embarked on an experiment to document the effects of a high sugar diet, on his once healthy body, consuming only foods commonly perceived as 'healthy'. Through his journey, Damon highlighted some of the issues in the sugar industry and shared where sugar lurks on supermarket shelves. We watched as he stacked on 'cheesecake' and his body started to get sick. It's a rather shocking documentary, but if you take the time to watch it – it will show you just how damaging sugar is to a human body and just *how quickly* it does that damage.

Slashing sugar

'But I love sugar,' I hear you confess. I did too. Weaning off sugar creates a mild depressive effect, which unfortunately enough can be easily fixed just by consuming more sugar (you've heard the term 'sugar fix').

Have you ever heard the term 'hangry'? I'm sure you have, but for those not familiar with the colloquialism, 'hangry' is when our body is depleted of glucose and it's looking for the next 'hit'. Hungry and angry.

Your body is experiencing withdrawal symptoms. When our body relies on glucose solely for fuel, it thinks it's running out of energy, because it isn't used to using the back-up source of fat. At the same time, insulin is high, because of excess blood sugar, preventing the use of this stored fat. So, it gets cross. Your body turns into a crabby, floor-rolling, foot stamping toddler, who (more often than not) wins, despite your best intentions and all the promises you made to yourself, when you finally succumb and stuff your favourite chocolate bar in your face.

Now you know about the negative impacts refined sugar can have on your body and mind, you can make better choices about the foods you choose. The first step is getting educated about where sugar lurks—believe it or not, a food needn't even taste all that sweet for it to be loaded with sugar and refined seed oils. When it comes to convenience and packaged foods, let the ingredients label be your guide, and be aware that just because something boasts that it's 'low-carb' or a 'diet' food doesn't mean it's free of sugar.

Sugar is hidden in the strangest places. That bottle of tomato sauce, buns and bread, common condiments, health food, cereal and canned foods. Stir fry, pizza and pasta sauces. Soft drinks, baked goods, lollies, flavoured milks, energy drinks and desserts can all have massively high amounts of sugar. Some foods have four or five kinds of sugar, tucked away neatly in the ingredients list under the guise of another tricky sounding name.

NAMES FOR HIDDEN SUGAR

Agave nectar	Dextrin	Maltol
Anhydrous dextrose	Dextrose	Maltose
Barbados sugar	Diastatic malt	Mannose
Barley malt	Diatase	Maple syrup
Barley malt syrup	Ethyl maltol	Molasses
Beet sugar	Evaporated cane juice	Muscovado
Brown sugar	Free-flowing brown sugars	Nectar
Buttered syrup	Fructose	Palm sugar
Cane juice	Fruit juice	Pancake syrup
Cane juice crystals	Fruit juice concentrate	Panela
Cane sugar	Galactose	Panocha
Caramel	Glucose	Powdered sugar
Carob syrup	Glucose syrup solids	Raw sugar
Castor sugar	Golden sugar	Refiner's syrup
Coconut palm sugar	Golden syrup	Rice syrup
Coconut sugar	Grape sugar	Saccharose
Confectioner's sugar	High-fructose corn syrup	Sorghum syrup
Corn sweetener	Honey	Sucrose
Corn syrup	Icing sugar	Sweet sorghum
Corn syrup solids	Isoglucose	Syrup
Crystalline fructose	Invert sugar	Table sugar
D-ribose	Lactose	Treacle
Date sugar	Malt	Turbinado sugar
Dehydrated cane juice	Malt syrup	White granulated sugar
Demerara sugar	Maltodextrin	Yellow sugar

Sugar is hidden in over eighty different names

Keep an eye out for some of the aliases sugar goes by, including dextrose, sucralose, high fructose corn syrup, agave syrup, fructose, cane crystals, maltodextrin, xylose and malt syrup. These are simply… sugar, causing the same blood sugar response. Unfortunately, food labelling laws mean you *do* need to be somewhat a sugar sleuth. Be aware that some juices labelled 'no added sugar' have more sugar in the form of fructose than a can of soft drink!

Is it any wonder we struggle?

98

Cutting back on added sugar: Don't start by trying to resist that cheesecake head-on. Cut it slowly using these tips.

- Replace sugary soft drinks, fruit juice and post workout or energy drinks with plain or sparkling water. Add a squeeze of lime, lemon or mint for extra flavour.
- Replace sugar with friendly sweeteners like monkfruit, erythritol and stevia that don't provoke a blood sugar response.
- Start your day the low-sugar way with filling protein or quality fats.
- Read labels and choose no-sugar options.
- Choose unsweetened snacks.
- Rethink dessert or find a lower-sugar version.
- Focus on healthy whole foods. Even nuts taste sweet when you're off sugar.
- Cravings are often a sign of dehydration or mineral deficiency. Have a glass of water and some pink salt.
- Replace sugar-filled food with satisfying berries and cream/yogurt or make a dessert from something naturally sweet, like coconut milk or cream (ideas in the sweet recipe section of this book).
- Take chromium.

Best of all, you'll save so much money.

Do:

Turn the packet of your favourite food over. Take a look at the amount of ingredients in your favourite foods. Is there hidden sugar in there? More than one kind? A bottle of BBQ sauce I picked up recently had no fewer than *four* types of sugar in the ingredients.

Less than five ingredients. A good rule of thumb when you're choosing a packaged product, is to make sure that there are fewer than five ingredients, and fewer than five grams of carbs per serving. Resisting the chips, cakes, or chocolate-covered almonds doesn't have to be a battle between willpower and craving.

Embrace new flavours. Processed foods are mostly based on sugar and the lethal combination of processed oils. Dress up meat or vegetables with other flavours—fats like butter and ghee, quality salt, homemade sauces, seasonal vegetables, cured meats, mushrooms, tomato paste, miso, soy sauce and hard-aged cheeses such as parmesan, along with herbs for adding hearty flavours. Over time, you'll notice your cravings start to diminish.

Find alternatives for high-bliss-point foods. We don't stop eating these kinds of foods when we're full due to our satiety hormone being flipped off—we stop only when this food in front of us runs out. Remember that block of chocolate? Use this knowledge to your advantage. Plug the words keto or low-carb, or no sugar in front of anything you're craving into google and grab the ingredients to make it at home.

Be prepared. Carry your favourite snack with you in your handbag or backpack—so you can head off cravings at the pass. A snack size, low carb option can mean the difference between a day of guilt or a day of freedom.

Go smaller. Acknowledge your caveman brain and set out a portion of your trigger foods. Try smaller individually-wrapped portions as we eat substantially less than if we're given the same total amount in a large size. Even if you go back for seconds (totally normal), you'll eat less than if you had the entire bag sitting in front of you.

Hydrate. Often hunger is mistaken for thirst. Drink a glass of water if you're starting to feel the urge to forage.

There are some amazing sugar-free desserts available for you in the recipes section of this book. Enjoy them!

CHAPTER 7

The goss on grain

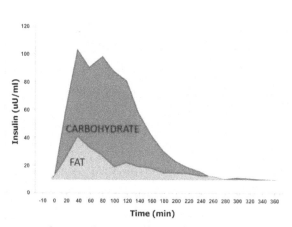

The Carb / Insulin Spike Graph

So far, you'd be forgiven for thinking that I believe carbs are The devil—they aren't. However, they are a potent insulin stimulator—in order to lose weight and improve our neural and metabolic health, we need to lower our insulin, and the easiest and most effective way is to lower our starchy carbohydrate intake.

Carbohydrates are complex sugars that provide energy. Molecules are strung together in long chains. Both simple and complex carbohydrates are turned to glucose (blood sugar) in the body and are used as energy. They both spike blood sugar and create an insulin response too. These are found in foods such as peas, corn, fruit, legumes, whole grains and root vegetables.

Currently, we get an average of almost 50 per cent of our energy intake from grains. Before agriculture, most human food sources were carbohydrate-poor, and many diets, particularly in the northern hemisphere, were high in fat. Before the industrial revolution, all human diets were absent of the highly refined grains that are mostly responsible today for the massive occurrence of obesity and type 2 diabetes.

Don't get me wrong. I love pasta and baked potatoes, especially slathered in butter, with melty cheese oozing over the sides. Yum! However, we can access better choice carbohydrates that *don't spike our blood sugar,* in above ground vegetables filled with healthy fibre such as cauliflower, broccoli, cucumbers, beans, cabbage, zucchini, eggplant and brussels sprouts.

For a printable list – just shoot me an email at lazyketones@gmail.com and I'll send it over. You might also like to check out my blog at https://tiny.one/foodweloveblog for more information on this. There's also a basic food list in Appendix A for you.

When we eat seasonal produce in conjunction with quality dietary fat, the body gets all fabulous and ships the essential vitamins and minerals from our food, to our cells on the express train—offering nutrition *and* satiety. Exit diet roundabout! It's also a heck of a lot cheaper than being a food slave and succumbing to last minute expensive impulse cravings at Donut King.

Humans first began eating grains about 75,000 years ago in western Asia. The ancestors of today's wheat, including einkorn and emmer, grew wild near the banks of rivers and people harvested the seeds and grasses that grew naturally near their communities.

Today, grain is widely available and a convenient diet staple thanks to our current food pyramid and technology of mass cultivation. We harvest seeds of grasses such as wheat, oats, rice and corn. These are the most common grains on our planet. You've already heard wheat is Australia's top export crop. Sorghum, millet, rye and barley are other important grains that we use to feed livestock and manufacture some cooking oils, fuels and cosmetics. We also make alcohol from them—some would say that's very important for their mental health! More on libation later. Much of world's grain supply is used in the manufacture of industrial products like biodiesel and ethanol, which also, interestingly can be made from corn.

Grains are very versatile, they can be turned into numerous things we love including bread, fried rice, donuts and pasta. They can be eaten fresh or stored for long periods. If your mouth is watering at these and you're worried about lowering carbs and missing your crusty loaf, check out the bread replacement recipes in the back—I promise you won't miss bread!

The preservation of flour became vitally important during the industrial revolution of the 1800s. Transportation methods and distance logistics were a challenge—grains didn't have a very long shelf life and the supplies were spoiling. Once grain is milled, the fatty acids oxidise and flour starts to turn rancid. The fatty acids of the germ react the moment they are exposed to oxygen. Back then, the information available on vitamins, micronutrients and amino acids, was relatively unexplored and removing the germ seemed like an effective solution for longevity. Without the germ, the flour didn't spoil.

The term 'refined' grain, in contrast to 'whole' grain, refers to grain products, like white flour, for example, that has been significantly milled and modified from its natural state. This process involves mechanically husking—removing the fibre and the nutrition dense outer bran from the germ, through selective sifting or grinding. Then, we further refine using industrial processes like bleaching and treating with a chemical called bromine. After that, crazily, we add back in what we took out—*essential*, naturally occurring minerals and vitamins like thiamine, riboflavin, niacin and iron.

The issue is that as we remove the fibre, we remove the mechanism that controls slow-release absorption into our blood stream. Again, a sugar spike, provoking high insulin response, high-fat storage signalling, and at the same time blocking fat release. We need insulin to process blood sugar. When you eat carbohydrates, you need insulin.

Insulin is a storage hormone.

You've been told that you need carbs. We do *not need* carbs.

In the 2005 textbook, *Dietary Reference Intakes for Energy,* the US Food and Nutrition Board states: '*The lower limit of dietary carbohydrate compatible with life apparently is zero, provided that adequate amounts of protein and fat are consumed.*' This information confirms that carbs aren't actually necessary.

Truly, you don't really need any carbs at all. They said you might die or waste away or your body might eat your muscles (sarcopenia) without carbs. Not true. It's just *simply* not the case. Your body can make glucose from protein, and it can make *any* glucose it needs from amino acids and glycerol found in fatty acids. This process is known as gluconeogenesis.

You don't even need carbohydrates for exercise. Your performance will be better in ketosis because of longer lasting energy, as we have witnessed with the French cycling team, who are utilising ketones as their secret weapon to gain a competitive advantage over their opponents.

You're saying '*Nooooooooooo, Emmmmmaaaaa, I can't do it!*'

But you can. I do understand your challenge—I used to be a carboholic. Pasta, bread, donuts—you name it, I was there! Front of the line and back for seconds.

As you've read, we had some kind of starchy carbs with almost every meal when I was a kid. However, once I reduced these in my diet and added fats like butter and olive oil, so I wasn't hungry, my waistline started shrinking because I wasn't food hunting and I minimised my insulin response. As I filled up on good fats, the cravings for sugar and fast energy food completely disappeared, because I was so satisfied and off the crazy coaster.

I rarely eat pies and donuts now, not because I can't (I'm not adverse to the odd steak, bacon and cheese pie), but because I don't crave them anymore. I recently found out I was gluten intolerant in my blood tests. Further research shows that over 80 per cent of the human race has some kind of gluten intolerance, ranging from celiac disease (an autoimmune response) to a couple of the four hereditary genes that are responsible for gluten intolerance. Yes, that's right—we inherit the genes! I had no idea! I think I was just used to feeling crumby (pardon the pun).

You can choose to discard this advice and put this book back on the shelf, but *what if* you tried just a few of these simple switches below, combined with tools for better choices and dramatically improved your health, brain and waistline? Who knows, you might even feel great?

Simple tips to avoid sending cheesecake straight to the storage shed:

- If you're making a roast, swap out starchy, below-the-ground root vegetables like carrots, beetroot, potato, for lower-carbohydrate options like baked cauliflower, leeks, eggplant, zucchini, roasted capsicum, and a side of gorgeous greens cooked in butter. We often have a slow-cooked leg of lamb or pork, cooked on a bed of celery, onion and leek, which also makes the best gravy! I've included the recipes at the back for you. You're welcome!

- Replace pasta and rice with lower-carb choices like zoodles (zucchini noodles), cabbage that is finely shredded and cooked with butter and spices. Try konjac or edamame noodles (you'll find them in the health food aisle), cauliflower rice and seasonal green veg.

- Blood sugar-friendly veggies—all types of lettuce, spinach and other seasonal greens are great options. Green vegetables tend to be lower in carbs than veggies with a lot of colour, but it's great to eat the rainbow. For example, green cabbage is lower in carbs than purple cabbage, so it prompts less of a blood sugar response. Green capsicums are also somewhat lower in carbs than red or yellow. Don't sweat this. Eat seasonal, eat fresh, eat local.

- Replace traditional grain flours such as:
almond flour, coconut flour, chia flour, flax meal, sunflower seed, pumpkin seed flour and psyllium husk.

PART 2.

The how to...

CHAPTER 8

The great undoing

> '*Things are created twice; first mentally, then physically. The key is to begin with the end in mind, with a vision and a blueprint of the desired result.*'
> STEPHEN R. COVEY

If what you've read makes sense so far, read on. If you are ready to reclaim your mood, your focus, your sleep, your mojo and make some changes, then let's do this. This is the *how* part of the book and here are some additional keys to unlock your doors.

Water

Even mild dehydration can affect everything from your skin to your gut health. Proper hydration is absolutely vital for promoting healthy digestion. Since dehydration can cause bowel issues among other things, hydration is super important—make sure you're getting enough fluid each day. Two to three litres is a good benchmark. You can tell if you're dehydrated by checking out your pee! It should be the colour of light lemonade, not yellow like apple juice.

Make water your go-to choice. Add mint, berries, lemon or lime for a fresh twist. If you reach for a sweet drink instead of a meal or snack when you're truly hungry, you're not likely to feel satisfied and may fill up on 'empty calories' and end up back on the rollercoaster. A glass of apple juice will leave you hungrier than the whole apple, as the juice is missing the vital fibre that slows down absorption into the blood. Skip it.

Eat your veggies

When you first start this lifestyle, the foods you're likely to stock (and fill) up on are non-starchy vegetables, like leafy greens, sprouts, cauliflower, broccoli and asparagus, avocado and mushrooms.

Remember too, not all vegetables are created equal when it comes to blood sugar response. Limit veggies high in starch, like potatoes and corn, these are best enjoyed in moderation until you reach your goals. They can be slowly re-introduced once you're metabolically flexible or even once a week, rather than all the time.

More healthy fat

I know your idea of a 'diet' is not usually 'eat more fat', but when you're reducing your carb intake, you get to boost your nutrition and satiety in other exciting ways—one of the most satisfying ways is to add healthy fats. Add macadamia, coconut or olive oil, butter, or ghee to your meals. Your brain will *love* you for it, as will your appetite—or more accurately—lack of impulsive appetite.

Pack in your protein

As you're adjusting your carb vs. fat intake, don't forget about the powerful punch of protein-rich foods like eggs, chia seeds, yogurt, cheese, nuts and seeds, meat, poultry and full-fat dairy—these will help you feel full and offer many additional health benefits as well. Many sources of protein are also rich in amino acids, antioxidants and other essential nutrients. Great for your brain and mood too.

Portion proportion

Try eating off smaller plates—start with healthy fats and protein combos to get your tummy juices flowing—this aids with digestion, then consume your veg.

Food cravings

If you're struggling with combatting cravings—firstly, check your water intake—are you dehydrated? Secondly, have you been eating enough colours? Cravings can be caused by deficiencies in micronutrients. You may also need to add in some pink salt or even supplement with magnesium and potassium, sodium or spirulina. Take one-eighth of a teaspoon of pink salt and suck it, mix it in water or shot it in a glass—it doesn't matter how you do it, just try it! Especially if you have a headache or a foggy brain. I've also added a cravings cheat sheet for you in Appendix A, page 237.

Indulge

Yes, you read that correctly. The feeling of deprivation is responsible for many 'diet fails'. When you do have a treat, have something you *really* enjoy. Even better, google a keto or low-carb friendly version of the treat. You'll feel more satisfied having a small slice of delicious keto friendly cheesecake, (I just happened to pop the one from the front cover in the recipe section for you)—than if you're tempted to binge on the donuts, which as you have learned, are a lethal combo of refined oils and bleached flours. Remember, good fats are filling. Oxidised oils are damaging. Guilt is just as detrimental to your journey and can sabotage fat loss by causing a stress and store response, so have the treat—and enjoy it.

Ketones

You can also try using natural bio-identical ketones (my suggestion Appendix B), which helped me hack ketosis and fat-burning, plus killed my cravings fast—currently the only naturally fermented ones on the market. Natural ketones are truly a such fabulous tool and changed my life. If you're using ketones, *please* make sure they are bioidentical, otherwise it's just more rubbish your body needs to clean up and flush out.

Recently there have been heaps of interesting studies around bioidentical natural ketones. In one particular study, researchers from Mass General Hospital studied young adults using specialised MRIs. They scanned the brains of their healthy volunteers—firstly, after following a SAD (Standard American/Australian Cardboard Diet), again after a 12-hour fasting period, and, for a third time, a week later—after the subjects followed a keto-style diet. This was followed by another randomised trial, where the brains of healthy volunteers were scanned firstly after consuming their standard diet, again after a 12-hour fast, and yet again after breaking their fast with a glucose dosage. Then again, breaking their fast with the same natural bio-identical exogenous ketone drink I used to kickstart my fat loss.

These researchers found that the keto diet, drinking these particular ketones and intermittent fasting all helped *equally to improve the stability* of brain networks, and used in trifecta, are a powerful catalyst for ketosis activation. So, it doesn't matter how you get ketones in your system, via a drink, fasting or via a strict keto diet, the *same* benefits apply and can amplify your results.

This is in direct contrast to the SAD 'cardboard 'diet which actually *destabilised* the brain. These pioneer researchers also showed that these ketones further improved stability *even when combined* with glucose. Pretty cool, huh? If you have difficulty following and staying on a ketogenic diet you may like to consider adding these exogenous ketones to your day and becoming a dual-fuelled bio-hacked, optimised human. For more info on these, shoot me an email at lazyketones@gmail.com.

The best 'diet' of all? The one you will stick to.

It's a process

Processed food is so ingrained in our everyday eating, yet modern society has witnessed an alarming increase in obesity, type 2 diabetes and many other diseases associated with our current food pyramid and lifestyle. Instead of preserving meats with salts and using a traditional curing process, we add preservatives with numbers! Try to avoid anything in an ingredient list that has numbers, or ingredients you can't read. Whenever possible, *avoid* ready-to-serve, additive heavy food. Head towards healthier food choices with less ingredients or home-cooked meals from seasonal produce. Five or fewer ingredients is a good aim.

Have you ever seen the image of the McDonald's sandwich that never becomes mouldy? By contrast, our fresh food seems to spoil rather quickly. Unfortunately, preservatives in our food are also culprits in the deterioration of our health globally.

Our guts and brains are intrinsically linked through the Vegas nerve. Your tummy flora is highly relevant when it comes to brain and body health. Emulsifiers, thickeners, and preservatives have effects on this colony in our gut and likewise on the cells of the immune system too. Emulsifiers are detergent-like molecules used by the food industry as stabilisers for processed foods. These significantly impact us through disruption of the gut flora, leading to increased impulse food intake (among other things) which, in turn, drives obesity by increasing fat mass and storage. As well as contributing to excessive fat mass accumulation, emulsifiers and stabilising additives are associated with low-grade inflammation, which also plays a crucial role in the onset of obesity and related metabolic disorders.

What is inflammation?

Processed foods contain sugar and other chemicals that result in oxidation. When the body processes sugar, excess additives or complex carbohydrates, it simultaneously creates oxidation—the more we consume, the more oxidation our body has to deal with.

Oxidation produces free radicals—molecules that interact within our cells, resulting in cellular stress and damage. Free radicals are necessary and normal as they also stimulate repair, however, when an excess of free radicals is produced, the repair processes are overwhelmed—this becomes an issue and is called oxidative stress. It can cause eyesight issues, ageing, grey hair, wrinkles, arthritis and even cancer. This is *just* what is visually apparent.

Five tips to age gracefully
- Reduce sugar, complex refined carbs and processed foods.
- Get plenty of sleep—essential for rejuvenation.
- De-stress—go for a walk, rest, enjoy nature, catch up with friends, read a good book, garden or go to the beach.
- Practise gratitude—it *literally* re-wires your brain and it's impossible to feel grumpy, if you're in a state of gratefulness.
- Avoid toxins and additives where possible such as cigarettes, sugars, food additives and preservatives, exhaust fumes, certain plastics. If fat loss is a goal—it might be worth considering lowering alcohol too. More on that later.

CHAPTER 9

You are not a tree

Life is a spiderweb and we are all connected. Never underestimate the ripple you can create if you spread a little love to each and every person you run into every day? What if your smile and friendly greeting has a positive impact on the cashier at the supermarket and she goes home to her kids in a happier mood? What about the jogger or bushwalker you walk past? If you throw out a smile as you pass, you just never know what impact you can have on that person, and in the process feel better about yourself too. A little gratitude goes a *very* long way. Gratefulness and smiling creates endorphins, the 'feel-goods', and believe it or not, can help you on your journey to a happier and healthier you.

Imagine if you paid for the coffee of the person behind you in the drive through? How would that impact their day? And the best bit is that you get to feel good knowing you made someone smile and feel pretty damn awesome about it. Give it a try.

In contrast, think about how you impact your friends, colleagues or family when you come home in a bad mood? Is it contagious? Yes, it is. Bring the light, let go of the dark. I know this seems too silly and basic for words, yet this *alone* can impact your health tremendously. You can choose your own weather. It sounds cliché, but *be the sunshine, not the storm.* Grateful, happy people live longer too!

Next time you're at the traffic lights in your car, or sitting on a bus, train or plane, *I dare you* to give a big cheesy smile at someone, even if they aren't watching. Look at what happens when they feel the energy from your smile. They will either look up and return the smile, or they will look away hurriedly, but either way, you'll have impacted them in some positive way. It's a ripple effect.

Little things for great minds

- **Attitude of gratitude.** Do you believe you can? Say it: '*I can,*' and '*If she can do it, I can do it.*' Starting the day with an attitude of gratitude and belief (even when you don't believe it) is proven to switch on endorphins, the feel-good chemistry in our brain. I often start my day with a '*you've got this*' in the mirror. Actually, it's more like, '*You are magnificent, Emma,*' but that's another tale for another day. Think about *who* and *what* you are grateful for, daily.

- **Be careful with concrete**. You are not a tree. You are not stuck. This is *your* life and *your* brain health, and you can make any change *any time* you damn well want to.

- **Forgive yourself**. If fat loss is a goal and you trip over, maybe you ate the whole packet of chips, or an ice-cream accidentally fell in your mouth, please don't sweat it. Instead of beating yourself up, get busy finding a low-carb, non-insulin spiking substitute for next time. Look for the lesson, find the blessing and move on.

- **Be mindful**. This is a little like the attitude of gratitude, with a twist. Take time to plant your feet on the grass, connect to the earth, breathe and even meditate. Go for a 20-minute walk. Stress in our current world is so high and our cortisol is on overdrive—this can also lead to your body holding on to fat as a safety mechanism. You've heard of fight or flight? This can break the habit for you, by letting your body know it's safe.

- **Weight**. Those stupid measurement platforms we stand on in the bathroom can't be trusted. The scales *lie*. Weight is almost irrelevant, despite what you've been told. You can lose 'weight' in the form of water, fat or muscle. A kilogram of fat and a kilogram of muscle are different in volume, and therefore size. A better way to benchmark is hip-to-waist ratio.

There are many factors like water retention and hormones at play here. As you improve your body composition and lose fat, you may not see the scales change, but you will feel your pants get lose. Find time to take 'before' measurements – you'll be so glad you did, and photos too, if fat loss is a goal for you. If you *must* weigh yourself—make it only once a month, *not* every single day because *that is called sabotage*. A kilogram of muscle and a kilogram of fat are *not* the same thing. I want you to trust the way you feel. This may not make sense now, but it will.

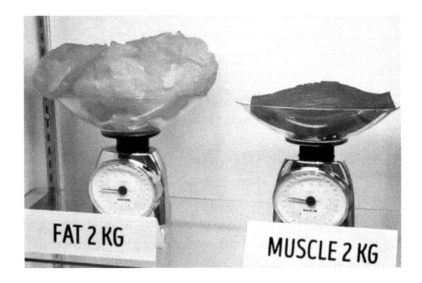

- **How are the feels?** If it's not fat loss you're chasing— take note of how you feel. Take a mental snapshot of your mood, sleep, cravings, energy and brain clarity, and even better, write it down. These are very useful benchmarks as you move forward.

- **Time.** It is unbelievably important that you give your healing enough time to occur. There is much *undoing* to take place inside your body and brain. You may not always see the results immediately. We didn't get here overnight. Be gentle on you.

- **Minimise stress**. Stress causes the production of cortisol and cortisol signals to your body that this is a fight or flight situation—it signals to your parasympathetic nervous system that you might die while getting back to your cave. Stress puts your adrenals into overdrive. Breathe, take a walk and put the phone down first thing in the morning and late at night. Be present. Enjoy your kids, pets and partner—not necessarily in that order!

124

- **Comparison is the thief of joy**. My journey at times has been frustrating. Some days, it's one step forward and two steps back. Everyone is so different, and you cannot compare your results with anybody else's. Some people will drop weight faster than a balloon losing air—it seemingly melts off their body overnight, while for others it may take longer. Don't give up on your *long-term health* because of comparison to others or lack of instant 'results'.

- **Internal clean up**. Your body may experience a detox. When we eat processed foods and ingest toxins that our body doesn't know what to do with, it swaddles them protectively in the security of our fat, (particularly around our middle), to make sure what isn't healthy for us, can't do too much damage. As you start to release the contents of fat cells, you may experience a 'cleaning out' of these toxins. This is essential. Keep your water up and take a little pink salt or a sugar free electrolyte to replace essential minerals you lose. Spirulina can be a helpful supplement to help remove toxins.

- **Hydration**. If you don't drink enough water, your body struggles to release these toxins and it will re-store them protectively in your cheesecake (read: storage mode). It also can't connect the dots in your brain, leading to brain fog and fatigue if you're dehydrated.

- **Water retention.** Did you know that as you lose 'weight', you may hold onto water? Often when you start a new lifestyle, your body retains fluid because it isn't quite sure what it's going to have to deal with, and it's a bit of a safety net. In order to process glucose, you need quite a lot of water. When you lower carbohydrates, your body will hold onto that water 'just in case', resulting in bloating. Now, I don't know about you, but I can put on a couple of kilograms within a couple of hours, then lose it that same day. Once your body knows it's not going to die, it will release it, resulting in what is often called 'the whoosh' effect.

- **Hormones**—more on this in the next chapter. Suffice to say they are so relevant to your journey, they get a whole chapter. Some of the most important hormones with regard to fat loss are insulin, cortisol, adrenalin, ghrelin and leptin.

- **Learn**. Educate yourself. Listen to podcasts like *Low Carb MD* and *Low Carb Down-Under* and build your knowledge. I also love Robb Wolfe, Dr Jason Fung, Dr Eric Berg, BU with Brian Underwood podcast, and the website *Diet Doctor*. Watch the documentaries *The Magic Pill* and *That Sugar Film* and get educated. Well intentioned friends and family probably won't understand what you're doing. They really only want to look after you, however some may even be threatened by your forward momentum. They may be a little jealous and unwittingly sabotage you. Remember that they are still stuck in the diet hypothesis loop. Just thank them for caring and take a big step over their advice. Remember health professionals too, may fall into this category, so work with one who understands. Your friends will ask about your lifestyle when they are ready. Who doesn't want to eat the yummiest food ever and to feel awesome—just saying.

- **Sleep is a weapon**. When you're tired, your body wants you to feed it. It demands energy, and fast energy, and it will upregulate your hunger hormones to make sure you hunt for food. You literally have *no* will power. Make sure you're getting at least seven to eight hours of sleep a night, so your body is repaired and happy.

- **Don't drink your calories**. Look for alternatives. If you need a flavoured drink, try mixing half a glass of soda water or mineral water with your bevvy of choice.

- **Night needs.** Aim not to have high-carbohydrate foods, especially first thing in the morning and late at night. Read: blood sugar response and hello carb-and-crash cycle. Try not to eat after 8 pm. Give your digestion a rest.

- **Intermittent fasting** also rests your digestion, triggers cell regeneration and prompts a clean-up of damaged and defective cells. I've explained this more thoroughly in the next chapter.

- **Calorie counting**—it isn't necessary to count your calories. We can introduce macro tracking later if your body isn't playing nicely at letting go of its winter storage. It is equally important to be eating enough. I've put some details about our tips group and one on one coaching options available to you in the back of this book, if you need a little more help or accountability.

- **Keep going**. Get back on if you fall off. This is not a race, and you are not a tree.

CHAPTER 10

Hidden keys

O*ur bodies hate change.* One of the most important things to understand about successful and sustainable fat loss is that your body's storage 'thermostat' is preset and, as we all know, doesn't like giving back its energy reserves.

In his book, *The Obesity Code*, Dr Jason Fung describes body set weight in terms of air-conditioning in a house. The aircon is set to a particular comfortable room temperature. In summer, when it's hot outside, the thermostat turns on the air con to bring down the temperature of the room. In winter, it also detects that the temperature is too cold, and it boosts the heat to the desired temperature, so your house stays at the perfect comfort level, due to the actions of the air con.

In our bodies, we have similar thermostats for body fat storage that are survival mechanisms. Our body tries very hard to maintain its preferred set weight, acting just like an air con unit. This is in direct contradiction to the 'calories in, calories out' hypothesis— this philosophy does not consider satiety, hormones or any other physiological signalling. If you deliberately overeat, your body tries to burn it off, then stores the rest, clever thing that it is.

We also have multiple overlapping satiety triggers to stop us from overeating. Satiety hormones such as leptin and the stretch receptors in our stomachs signal when we are too full, and stop us from eating too much, although if you've ever indulged at a Sizzler salad bar, you'll understand why these receptors can be a bit broken and even ignored. Sugar bypasses these important physiological mechanisms. On the flip side, ghrelin our hunger hormone is activated when we are hungry, tired or stressed.

Think about the time you ate too much at the buffet. You may have filled up on the fast fuel like bread and pasta. However, if we choose foods with higher fat or protein content, we are fuller faster, because our satiety hormones like leptin activate. Would you *really* be able to eat two more big steaks at the buffet, just because they were available? Gosh, no! I know I can *easily* fit in another caramel slice or three though. It is really, really hard to keep eating once we're full of the *right* food.

This primal satiety mechanism in our body makes so much sense. We are designed to stay within certain body-fat bookmarks. Too skinny, with no reserves and we die during the hard times (winter). Too fat, we can't catch the food we need to survive and may even get eaten by the meal instead. Wild animals rarely become obese, do they? Where are the really fat fish and obese antelope? Chubby lions? When food is plentiful, *numbers* of animals increase, instead of the *size* of the animal itself increasing. All wild animal populations share this effect.

The idea of 'a calorie is a calorie' has been pushed by Big Food trying to convince you that it is fine to swap 100 calories of avocado for 100 calories of Coca-Cola. This is all fine and dandy, except that the coke spikes your blood sugar and promotes insulin release and fat storage, and the avocado doesn't. As long as they keep people believing, Big Food can sell sugar and mega-processed foods and *still* tell people that 100 calories of spinach is as fattening as 100 calories of sugar. Hmmm, of course it isn't.

No wonder we are confused.

Obesity, as we have learned, is caused by excessive insulin, *not* too many calories. *Obesity is a hormonal imbalance.*

You might like to check out *The Obesity Code* by Dr Jason Fung. This is one of the books that changed my relationship with food. He also co-wrote one of my other favourite books called *The Fasting Lane.* Another great read regarding this topic is *Wired to Eat* by Robb Wolfe.

The hidden keys

If you've ever burst into tears at something as random as watching a corny advertisement or a Disney movie, you'll know that your hormones are at play. One of the magical things about this lifestyle is that it is also capable of balancing your hormones leading to better mood, sleep and less raving banshee moments.

Other hormones that can dramatically affect your wellbeing are:

Cortisol

Cortisol is our stress hormone and a leading lady in metabolism dysfunction. Cortisol has many roles in the human body, including balancing stress response, regulating metabolism and inflammatory response, plus *very importantly*—immune function. Cortisol receptors are found almost everywhere in the body, so this hormone is able to readily impact nearly every organ. This includes our nervous system, the respiratory and cardiovascular systems, our 'sexytime' system and our muscles.

Cortisol is a bestie with insulin, which as you'll remember, controls our blood sugar and can also kick you out of ketosis, as it stimulates blood sugar release. These two friends are regularly seen on dates together in your body. One of the roles of Cortisol is to stimulate fat and carbohydrate metabolism for fast energy—it's the 'fight or flight' response thing again.

When cortisol rises for extended periods of time, it can also cause resistance to insulin. Sometimes this can be reflected in an increase in appetite and can cause cravings for sweet, high-fat and salty foods. See the cheat sheet for what your cravings mean and how you can hack them in Appendix A.

Cortisol also tells your brain you're under threat. If that threat continues to appear, it signals to your body to fill the fat cells near the liver (near your tummy) in case food becomes scarce or you need a fast get away.

To add insult to injury, those fat cells in your belly also contain *more* cortisol receptors which can make *more* cortisol, so it's a double-edged sword, and a vicious circle.

Strategies for combat

There are many effective methods to help reduce cortisol levels and troubleshoot possible cortisol related weight gain. The most effective strategies include:

- Thoughtful rather than crazy mad exercise.
- Mindful eating (being present—this is why sitting at the table to eat is beneficial).
- Getting plenty of good quality sleep.
- Doing things you enjoy to wind down. I like to get in the garden and pull weeds or hang with my chooks. Go for a walk on the beach, birdwatch or read a book. Listen to your favourite music or a podcast.
- Practicing meditation and gratefulness is a wonderful technique for stress reduction. It's impossible to be stressed when you're being grateful.
- Breathing—that's why your smart watch tells you to breathe. That's also why it's called a smart watch. It knows you're stressed. Breathing slowly sends a message to the para-sympathetic nervous system to tell your body that you're just fine thank you very much, and it doesn't need to worry about you.

Dopamine

Dopamine is a messenger—a neurotransmitter that our nervous system uses to communicate between cells. This chemical courier plays a huge role in how we feel pleasure. It's part of our unique human ability to think and plan. Not enough dopamine can leave us with cravings, while too much can cause addictive behaviours. Remember my happy Sunday afternoon thoughts with my grandma and ice-cream? Even the memories of this time flood me with dopamine. FYI—the same is true of feeling and remembering fear and simultaneous cortisol release.

Activities like dancing, walking, a trip to the beach or the mountains or treating yourself to a massage are wonderful creators of dopamine in our bodies. Do you need a better reason to visit the day spa or have a coffee with a friend?

Adrenaline

Adrenaline increases your heart rate, elevates your blood pressure and boosts energy supplies. Adrenaline, along with its pal, norepinephrine, is responsible for the immediate reaction we feel when stressed. If someone jumps out at you from behind a door and you get a fright—your heart is pounding. That message you got from a hater. The sight of your ex with another person. That's adrenaline. Also known as *fight or flight*. Along with the increase in heart rate, adrenaline focuses you and gives you a surge of energy—which biologically we needed to run away from a life-threatening situation. Your muscles are tense, your breathing gets faster, and you may get sweaty. Its rightly known as the *fight or flight* hormone and is useful for your protection—we also feel this, if we are outside our comfort zone. Stored energy is released, but if it isn't used to escape from the predator, it has to be re-stored.

Guess what its stored as?

The F-word. *Fat.*

How do we calm the farm?

Minimising blood sugar spikes reassure your body that you're not in crisis and you're not going to die at the hands of the neighbouring tribe.

- Eating nutrient dense, real foods.
- Try to minimise sugar.
- Give preference to lower fructose fruits such as berries or nuts.

Food allergies can also create an adrenal response. Common intolerances include wheat, soy, dairy, corn and eggs. If you suspect this is the case, you can try eliminating them and gradually re-introducing them one by one to see where the issue is.

Ghrelin

Ghrelin is the hunger hormone—it stimulates appetite and drives us to increase food intake. You can remember ghrelin because of *grrrrrrrr* (tummy growling noise) and it's responsible for turning on our hunger signals. It's produced in the gastrointestinal tract, particularly the stomach and is at the highest before a meal, returning to lower levels after mealtimes. Ghrelin also stimulates the brain, leading to an increase in appetite. It slows metabolism and decreases the body's ability to burn fat—because when you're eating, you're in 'storage mode'.

Leptin

Leptin is the yin to the yang of ghrelin. Leptin is our satiety hormone. Its job is to regulate fat storage compared to how much you eat and how much you burn. Leptin is produced by your body's fat cells. The more body fat you carry, the more leptin you produce. This is our biological mechanism to regulate body fat. The main function of leptin is to send a signal to your brain to communicate how much fat is stored in your fat cells, therefore balancing release of ghrelin. Leptin tells our brain that we have stores of energy and that we don't need any more food. But, unfortunately, with most of us eating carbs and sugars regularly, it's broken because those foods bypass the satiety mechanism.

Leptin resistance is a hormonal imbalance, and it makes losing weight even more challenging. Leptin resistance occurs when the cells in the brain stop recognising leptin's signals. When the cells are hungry, the brain doesn't perceive that food has entered and thinks that there's a famine coming. At this point, the brain turns on *all the hunger signals* and everything you eat goes straight to fat storage, without being used for energy, compounding the issue. If you suspect this is you, dropping your carbs and increasing your dietary fats should help to re-activate your leptin by turning on the satiety signal.

Inflammation

Although not a hormone, chronic inflammation causes many challenges in the human body, including dulling the brain's leptin receptors.

Some inflammatory culprits are:

- sugar
- seed oils
- alcohol

- processed meats
- gluten
- food additives
- dairy
- refined grains

Lowering inflammation is one of the healthiest things you can do to improve your body and immune system.

Does this all seem too big? In the next chapter, I'd like to teach you how to eat an elephant...

CHAPTER 11

How do you eat an elephant?

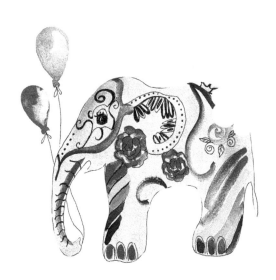

Exactly how do you eat an elephant?

Well, that's easy. One bite at a time.

By now I hope you've absorbed lots of tips and have a better idea of *where on earth* to start and that you're not too confused. I know it seems big. It truly isn't. It is about little steps to big changes. Choose just *one thing* a week to focus on, eat the elephant one bite at a time.

Let's put all these pieces together, now that we know this lifestyle isn't going to kill us, but rather, help heal us.

What are keto and low-carb?

Keto is not scary, and it's *not* going to kill you. It's really about cleaning up your diet and moving towards fresh, healthy, seasonal foods and minimising sugar, excess refined carbohydrates, packaged foods, preservatives and additives.

It's about *minimising the blood sugar response*. Teach yourself to think of it like this and you'll never have to follow another diet, ever.

When following a keto lifestyle, the bulk of your daily intake will come from dietary fat (roughly 70 per cent), moderate protein (20-30 per cent) and the rest in 'net' carbs per day. Net carbs are total carbohydrates less fibre.

Lowering your carbohydrate intake sufficiently also puts your body into the metabolic state of ketosis, the state we have spoken about, where you burn fat, in the absence of glucose, for fuel. The benefit of this primarily comes from lowering insulin by eating a succulent grass-fed steak smothered in butter with fresh vegetables or a bun-less cheeseburger and a side of greens, or a cauliflower cheese bake, even a delicious pizza made with alternative ingredients, rather than refined sugars and flours.

To activate ketosis, most people on keto stick to a range of 20–30 grams of carbs a day, mostly coming from greens.

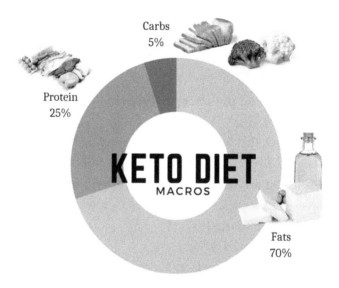

Carbs 5%

Protein 25%

KETO DIET
MACROS

Fats 70%

Types of keto

Dirty keto—eat whatever you want, regardless of ingredient quality and track macros (short for macronutrients). This version of the high-fat, low-carb ketogenic diet, is where you eat a mix of clean foods, fast foods, sugar-free drinks and processed snacks that fit into a specific set of macros. This style of eating is more flexible, however, there are some very good reasons, as we have read, to prioritise clean nutrient-dense whole foods whenever possible.

Some common *dirty keto* foods include:

- processed cheeses
- sugar-free soft drinks
- bun-less fast-food burgers
- pre-packaged meats
- pork rinds
- margarine and vegetable oils
- mayonnaise made with vegetable oils
- cheese crisps and other ultra-processed snacks
- sugar replacements
- tea and coffee
- keto bars and pre-packaged snacks

Lazy keto. I love this because strictly counting macros feels like a 'diet' to me and I reckon I'm more likely to fall off if I 'can't have' something. If you are the same, this is a great place to start. Lazy keto involves following keto guidelines to lower carb intake, but prioritising ingredient quality.

Some common *lazy keto* foods include:

- full-fat dairy
- no processed foods in boxes
- clear or sparkling water
- home-made beef hamburgers minus the bun
- quality steaks and chops with fat on
- leafy green salads or vegetables with olive oil as a dressing
- eggs and poultry
- quality fats like coconut and olive, avocado, ghee, butter.
- sugar replacements like monkfruit, stevia or erythritol
- fish and shellfish
- green vegetables

- berries
- nuts and seeds
- flours from nuts like almond flour and coconut flour
- coffee—with or without added fats—and tea

Clean keto involves prioritising whole, clean foods while sticking to your regular keto macronutrient breakdown. *Clean keto*, like lazy keto, is more about food quality, choosing clean, grass-fed, seasonal, pasture-raised and organic as often as possible.

Some common *clean keto* foods include:

- pasture-raised full-fat dairy
- clear or sparkling filtered water
- grass-fed meats and poultry
- leafy green organic salads with olive oil as a dressing
- eggs
- quality fats like coconut and olive, avocado, ghee, butter.
- minimal sugar replacements
- fish and seafood
- green leafy vegetables
- berries
- nuts and seeds
- unpackaged food
- tea or coffee with added clean fats.

Low-carb. Anything under 100–150 grams per day is generally considered compliant. This amount is *way* less than the standard western diet. You can achieve great results within this carbohydrate range, as long as you consume unprocessed, real foods.

You can see by all of these alternatives, it's really about eating clean food to satiety, and getting in where you fit in. Remember, the best lifestyle is the one you'll stick to. I follow a mix of these styles depending on the season, how busy I am and our budget.

Some simple changes will make a massive difference to the longevity and success of your journey, so here are my top tips on how to start. Also, you might like to check out the starter shopping list and pantry clean-up guide in Appendix A.

To do:

- Clean out your pantry.
- Toss vegetable oils. Replace with quality fats.
- Toss refined flour. Replace with nut flours.
- Throw out your low-fat dairy that's full of sugar and replace it with full-fat versions.
- Check labels on food and look for hidden sugar.
- If it's in a box, *really* have a think about if it's going to add or subtract to your health goals. Will it spike your blood sugar? If yes—toss it or donate it.
- Shop the outside of the aisles, buy seasonal and fresh.
- Snack on eggs, olives, cheese, fish, veg and salads, nuts, jerky, fresh salads with home-made dressing or mayo and little amounts of berries. For a free snack list please contact me and I'll send it through. Alternatively, you can google keto snacks or check out the recipes section in the back.
- Buy fattier cuts of meat. They are filling as well as being cheaper.
- Hydrate—staying hydrated is a key. We are mostly water and need to be topped up.

Swaps and substitutes

One of the simplest steps is to substitute to lower-carb alternatives. Follow these tips throughout the day:

- Start your day with coffee or water. Ditch milk for cream or sugar free nut milk.
- Swap bread for a low-carb wrap or use lettuce. At time of writing, some supermarkets have good low-carb bread options—remember though, just because it says low-carb, it doesn't mean it is. Check your labels. Under 5 grams of carbs a serving is a good aim.
- Reach for nuts, berries or a low-carb protein bar instead of hitting the food slot machine and keep a spare in your bag so you don't get caught out. (Watch out for maltitol in these – this can cause massive gut issues and quick loo runs).
- For dinner, cook up some spaghetti squash, cauliflower rice or zoodles instead of pasta.
- Snack on a pack of nuts, pork crackles or beef jerky instead of lollies or popcorn at the movies. Our local South African shop has marvellous droëwors, so this is often a go-to snack for our family.

Use tools

If you've hit a weight loss plateau, having all the information in front of you can help you to find a solution. Even if weight loss isn't your ultimate goal, keeping track of what and how much you eat can be very helpful, even for a week or so. Guessing or estimating portion sizes or nutritional information can easily get you off track and sabotage you. There are many apps and tools that will let you track your macronutrients for free.

Low-carb or keto with a family

As you embrace this new way of eating, your family might resist your efforts. I'd encourage you to share your goals with them. Tell them why this is important to you.

When I started this lifestyle, I still made my spaghetti bolognese sauce, for example, and instead of the pasta my family ate, I'd make zoodles (zucchini noodles) or a buttery toasted cauliflower rice for myself. Instead of potatoes with a roast, I'd bake extra low-carb vegetables for me, drizzled in olive oil and pink salt. Eventually, as time has passed, they have all embraced this lifestyle and feel much better for it. Hannah's skin cleared up, her shape changed, and her teen mood is generally stable. We have a better relationship because we are both calmer. These days we enjoy roasts, slow cooker meals, fish or a protein with a good side dish of green seasonal vegetables cooked in butter or olive oil.

Find support

Change is not always easy. Adjusting to changes you make and staying motivated for the long haul, will be so much easier if people have your back. You may have a supportive partner, friends, or family, but it can also be helpful to find others who are going through the same process. Look for local support groups with like-minded people. We have a big group online—reach out if you'd love an invite to our community or to jump on my next coaching course. Many online groups or forums like ours exist—some of them let you link up your fitness apps and activity trackers with others for day-to-day support. A little healthy competition and accountability might be just your thing.

Time

One of the most important things as you adopt this change is to pay attention to *how* you feel. It's not unusual for the first few days or weeks to be uncomfortable mentally and physically. You may experience frustration as your energy levels initially dip. Your body may act like a toddler, screaming for its energy fix and punishing you for the change you've made. Give it some time and your body and mind will adjust. You may also experience gastrointestinal symptoms and appetite alteration. Please know *these are temporary*, and it *will* be worth it, however these may make you feel like giving up. *Please don't.* Pink salt and adequate hydration plus upping your good fats will often assist with these short-lived hurdles.

Your body's response will guide you and leave you clues about when it's time to add more activity, or reduce your carbs a bit more, or delve deeper into the pool of knowledge. Listen to what your body needs—honouring that will help you reach your personal best, and you will eventually thrive.

Green foods list—These foods are very keto friendly

- Meat and poultry
- Full fat dairy
- Fish and shellfish
- Olives
- Eggs
- Cheese
- Butter
- Dripping and lard
- Oils such as olive, avocado and coconut
- Avocados and berries

- Nuts and nut butters
- Seeds
- Green or white vegetables (non-starchy) like zucchini, cauliflower, brussels sprouts, cabbage, bok and pak choy, broccoli, leafy greens
- Salt, pepper, herbs, spices, garlic, mustard, olives, vinegars
- Beef jerky
- Pork crackles

Red foods list—AVOID—these foods are not keto-friendly

- Processed and low-fat foods
- Sugary drinks and juices
- Premade dressings and sauces (always check the labels)
- Starchy vegetables like potato and corn
- Most fruits, especially bananas, red apples, grapes, oranges and dried fruits
- Vegetable oils and margarines
- Cashews
- Legumes like chickpeas, lentils and beans
- Grains and grain products like traditional flour, bread, rice, cereals, pasta and popcorn
- All sugars like maple, agave syrup and coconut sugar

PART 3.

Level up...

CHAPTER 12

Unlocking the storage shed

• ● •

> *'Breakfast is the most important meal of the day.'*
> DR JOHN HARVEY KELLOGG

Have you heard this before? You probably had this drummed into you like I did. And, in turn, I drummed it into my kid. *I was wrong.*

Do you still believe breakfast is the most important meal of the day? No matter if you're sitting down to a stack of pancakes, a bowl of cereal, bacon and eggs, or Vegemite on toast, there's a good chance you start every day with breakfast. After all, we've been told many times that it's the most important meal of the day. Maybe you just grab a muesli bar and a giant-sized coffee on your way into work. Either way, you're doing the 'healthy thing' right? Or are you?

I'm not really a breaky person, so it was a relief to find out what my body already knew, and that was, that breakfast wasn't essential.

The food and drink we associate with breakfast have only become ingrained in our psyche, as part of a very deliberate effort to get us to change our breakfast habits. The breakfast statement above that we are all so familiar with, was nothing more than a clever marketing slogan, and a really good one at that. Dr John Kellogg and his side-kick James Jackson, coined this belief that still exists today—breakfast cereal was touted to *give good general health and well-being*, but there was also a very specific agenda. Dr Kellogg, first invented granola and then cornflakes, as part of a purist diet designed to suppress sexual desire and lead us away from sin. *Yes*, breakfast cereal was supposed to save us from masturbation. In addition to 'saving' us, Kellogg's, the ever growing food conglomerate, made a tidy USD $1.4 billion profit in 2019 purely off its cereals and convenience foods.

Cereals popularity as a breakfast food hasn't been for spiritual reasons or health benefits—the real advantage of breakfast cereal is convenience. Shake it into a bowl, add some skim milk and you're good to go. You're also good to spike your blood sugar first thing in the morning and stay on the craving train as your body burns through the sugars, stores some for later and wants more (read—decreased willpower).

Breakfast hasn't always been part of people's daily routine. It was actually socially and morally frowned upon to eat breakfast until about the 17th century, with the reformation of the church. In medieval England and Europe, eating at the start of the day was only a habit for early workers. As people worked more for employers, rather than on their own land, they had to work long, uninterrupted days, often without food. A hearty breakfast allowed them to work longer days in fields tending crops.

It was once thought a *sin* to eat too early, and eating before morning mass was generally frowned upon. Fasting always was, and still is in many countries, a religious observation, and breakfast literally means breaking one's fast.

Breakfast is *not* compulsory.

Maybe right now you're breathing a huge sigh of relief like I did, because if you're not a breaky eater, you're off the hook! On the other hand, maybe you love breakfast. That's ok too! Always do what suits you and your body will thank you, but can I suggest that you begin your day with something that *doesn't* spike your blood sugar and lead you back onto the rollercoaster.

One of the simplest things you can do to burn through stored fat, restore health and clean up on a cellular level, is add some timed fed and fasted periods. This may challenge some of your long-held beliefs and is called intermittent fasting.

The other F-word

Fasting is perhaps one of the oldest and most powerful dietary interventions imaginable. Most cultures in human history have included habitual fasts, across Buddhism, Christianity, Islam, Judaism, Taoism, Jainism and Hinduism. In these cultures, fasting can last for just a few hours or a month, depending on the occasion and the religion. Fasting has always been associated with the Christian season of Lent, Ramadan for Muslims, and many other cultures and religions around the world, fast throughout the year.

Some of the more favourable effects of fasting include lowering body mass and a clean-up of damaged cells plus many other beneficial effects on health-related conditions, including lowering blood pressure, increasing insulin sensitivity and managing oxidative stress.

The easiest way to think of it, is that your body fat is stored as energy and when you fast (don't eat), your body will simply 'eat' your fat for energy. Bonus! If we start eating as soon as we get out of bed and do not stop 'refeeding' until we sleep, we are always in a *fed* state. Our body does not burn our own fat in the fed state – this would be counter-productive to survival. In a 'fed' state, we have not given our body any time to burn the previously stored energy, before piling in more food.

When losing weight, we only need to increase the amount of time spent burning stored energy and lower the fed time period for almost immediate results. This gives the body permission to use its stored energy, by accessing body fat.

Intermittent fasting

Intermittent fasting is called 'an ancient secret' because it is one of the most powerful dietary interventions for weight loss, yet it has been mostly ignored by doctors and dietitians for a long time, until recently. Intermittent fasting involves cycling between eating and not eating and can provide massive health benefits. It is also very popular among low carb doctors to reverse insulin resistance.

When we don't eat, we are in a fasted state. Basically, anytime you are not eating, you are intermittently fasting. For example, you may fast between finishing dinner and until breakfast the next day, a period of approximately 12–14 hours. If you look at it that way, intermittent fasting is really just a part of everyday life. If you can stretch that fasted window out to 16 or 18 hours, you'll see enormous benefits like less cravings, balanced blood sugar and melted fat from the storage shed.

I'm not for one minute suggesting that you should stop yourself from eating to satiety, but if you can find a balance between *fast and feast*, you get to set alight that big firewood stash in the shed.

Rather than being some sort of cruel food depravation, Intermittent fasting can be part of everyday, normal life. People lose weight, lower their blood pressure, and their blood sugar improves as they adopt intermittent fasting, even without any other dietary changes. Studies in humans, across the board, have shown that IF is safe and *incredibly* effective.

Um... isn't that starvation? Nope.

Starvation is the *involuntary* absence of food for a long period of time.

Fasting is the voluntary abstinence of food consumption.

You allow your body to burn what it's been storing for you, for when food is scarce. (Aren't we lucky food is plentiful). When you fast, food is easily available, but you are making a choice *not* to stuff the donut in your face. This can be done for a few hours, a few days or—with medical supervision—even a week or more.

> *Remember the cycle? Eat food; produce insulin; store sugar; produce fat, close door of fat cell.*

The process also goes backwards—when we do not eat, insulin levels fall: no food, leads to decreased insulin, door open, resulting in burning stored sugar and fat.

Fasting is best undertaken by someone who is not underweight and has enough stored body fat to live off (my hand is up). Importantly, know there is *nothing* wrong with it. It is what our bodies are designed to do. That's what cats, dogs, bears, lions and chooks do. That's what *we* humans do. If you're eating every few hours your body constantly uses the incoming food as energy, instead of your body fat. You are in storage mode, and your body is saving it for a time when there is nothing to eat. We are cavemen, remember.

By fasting, you can also trigger autophagy, one of the healthiest things you can do for your body. Autophagy kicks in at roughly the 18-hour mark when fasting.

Yes, believe it or not, you *are* able to survive without stuffing a donut in your face every two hours. Obesity is not a calorie imbalance problem, but rather a gradual increase in the thermostat dial over time, due to high blood sugar and potential insulin resistance.

TIMELINE OF
FASTING

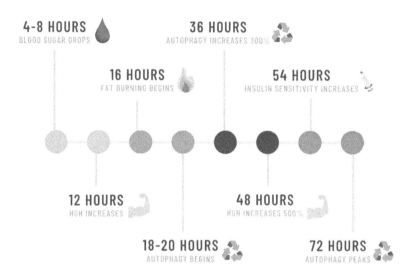

4-8 HOURS
BLOOD SUGAR DROPS

36 HOURS
AUTOPHAGY INCREASES 300%

16 HOURS
FAT BURNING BEGINS

54 HOURS
INSULIN SENSITIVITY INCREASES

12 HOURS
HGH INCREASES

48 HOURS
HGH INCREASES 500%

18-20 HOURS
AUTOPHAGY BEGINS

72 HOURS
AUTOPHAGY PEAKS

What is autophagy?

In 2016, the Nobel Prize in Physiology or Medicine was awarded to Yoshinori Ohsumi for his discovery of the mechanisms of autophagy.

The word autophagy comes from the Greek word auto (self) and phagein (to eat). This word, quite literally translated, means to *eat yourself.* Autophagy is the body's mechanism of cleaning up all the broken down, old cell machinery when there's not enough energy to keep it running efficiently. It is an efficient, orderly process that recycles cellular debris.

Dr Jason Fung uses this great analogy:

'Suppose you own a car. You love this car. You have great memories in it. You love to ride it. After a few years, it starts to look kind of beat up. After a few more, it's not looking so great. The car is costing you thousands of dollars every year to maintain. It's breaking down all the time.'

The same thing happens in our bodies. Cells become old and break down. This is called apoptosis, where cells are pre-destined to die. After a certain amount of time, you trade in the car, whether it's still working or not and get a new car. You don't have to worry about it breaking down on the highway.

Jason Fung continues: 'Is it better to keep the car around when it's nothing but a hunk of junk? Obviously not. So, you get rid of it and buy a snazzy new car.'

Autophagy means replacing old parts of the cell. Sometimes you don't need to replace the entire car. Sometimes, you just need to replace the battery. This happens in our cells too. Instead of killing off the whole cell (apoptosis), you only replace some of the cell components. This is the process of autophagy; meaning old cell membranes and cellular debris can be cleaned up by the body—reusing your car body, and replacing the working parts. For further reading on this, grab a copy of *The Fasting Lane*, by Dr Jason Fung, Eve Mayer and Megan Ramos.

Activation of autophagy

The key activator of autophagy is nutrient deprivation. In other words, fasting. When we don't eat, insulin goes down and glucagon goes up, stimulating autophagy. However, fasting is way more beneficial than just triggering autophagy.

Not only are we are clearing out all our old cellular gunk, fasting also *stimulates human growth hormone*. This signals our body to start producing some snazzy new bits like Stem cells. Stem cells are new cells that can be used to regenerate *any* part of the human body.

Fasting may also help to reverse the ageing process by replacing old cells—one of the reasons you see people who fast and follow keto looking so youthful.

Alternatively, keeping junky old defective cells is reflected in two of the main afflictions that plague the human race: Alzheimer's disease and cancer. Alzheimer's involves the accumulation of proteins that clog up the brain. Clinical trials are suggesting a process like autophagy has the ability to clear out old proteins and shows huge potential to be used in the prevention and treatment of brain issues such as Alzheimer's.

Benefits of timed eating
- activation of autophagy
- body fat/weight loss
- increased fat burning
- improved mental clarity and concentration
- increased energy
- increased human growth hormone (stem cells)
- lowered blood insulin
- lowered blood sugar levels
- reversing insulin resistance
- youthful appearance
- reduction of inflammation

How to turn off autophagy

Eat. Glucose and insulin turn off this important instinctual biological self-cleaning process. Autophagy is unique to fasting—it's not found in restricting calories or dieting.

Ways to fast

16:8 or 18:6
Pushing out your eating window just a little, is one of the easiest things you can do to make a huge impact. This involves a daily fasting window for 16–18 hours. This is also referred to, as a 6 or 8-hour eating 'window.' Eat all your meals within a time frame and fast for the rest of the day. You can do this daily or almost daily. For example, eat your meals between a time window of 12 pm to 8 pm. Usually, this means skipping breakfast. Some people prefer to skip dinner instead.

20:4
This is a 4-hour eating window, and a 20-hour fast. For example, you might eat in the 4 hours between 3 pm and 7 pm every day and fast for the other 20 hours. Usually, a large, quality meal or two smaller meals are consumed within this period.

OMAD or 24hr fast
'One meal a day' or OMAD involves fasting from dinnertime to dinnertime (or lunchtime to lunchtime). If you ate dinner on Monday, you would skip Tuesday's breakfast and lunch and eat dinner again that night. It is generally done one or two times a week.

5:2 fast
This fasting type involves five regular eating days and two fasting days. However, on these two fasting days, you are allowed to track

and eat 500 calories on each day. These calories can be consumed at any time during the day—either spread throughout the day or as a single meal. This is a version of intermittent fasting that Dr. Michael Mosley popularised in his book *The Fast Diet*. Personally, I'm not a fan because it would involve tracking and I'm lazy.

Alternate day fasting

Another approach to 5:2 is to have 'fasting days' where you eat 500 calories, not just twice a week, but every alternate day.

36-hour fasts

This involves fasting for the entire day and night. For example, if you eat dinner on Monday, you would fast all Tuesday and not eat again until breakfast Wednesday—36 hours of fasting. Knowing autophagy kicks in at 18 hours, this technique can kickstart a more powerful weight-loss benefit.

60-hour reboot

Once a month our community completes a coached 60-hour metabolic fast/reset. I once believed this was impossible. We use a bioidentical ketone kit to amplify the effect and stop cravings. Generally, we see losses of 2–3 centimetres across many parts of the body on completion of this program, but more importantly, we see clarity, focus and improvements in sleep and cravings, plus the amazing benefits of autophagy. I've put more information in Appendix B for you, if you want to investigate this as an amplifier.

Extended fasting

The first rule of extended fasts is to always check with your health care provider to ensure you are not at risk for fasting complications.

You shouldn't do intermittent fasting without supervision if you:

- are underweight
- have an eating disorder like anorexia or bulimia
- are pregnant
- are breastfeeding
- are under 18—you need extra nutrients to grow

You can fast under medical supervision if you:

- have type 1 diabetes
- take prescription medication
- have gout or high uric acid
- have any serious medical conditions, such as liver disease, kidney disease, or heart disease

Be aware that some doctors don't truly understand these benefits. They are seeing through the same set of eyes you previously have. Look until you find one who will work with you.

Frequently asked questions

Will intermittent fasting put me into starvation mode?
No. This is a common myth but it's not true. Some studies indicate that intermittent fasting may increase your metabolic rate and that it can improve overall body composition.

Can you exercise and fast at the same time?
Yes. You do not need to eat before exercise—instead, allow your body to burn your body fat for fuel. Whilst fasting, the body breaks down glycogen into glucose for energy. After that, the body increases body fat breakdown to provide energy. The body does not burn its own muscle

for energy unless it is forced to. This would not make evolutionary sense. It is important that you hydrate and replenish sodium.

Are there side effects?

Hunger is the most common side effect of intermittent fasting. This is less of an issue if you're already fat adapted. Hunger usually passes like a wave, so if you ignore it and drink a cup of tea or coffee or a glass of water, it will pass. Hunger will often increase into day two, as you use up your glycogen stores until you produce ketones to tap into your stored body fat. After that, hunger will gradually recede—as your body is now being powered by fat. In essence, your body is 'eating' its own fat for meals and is no longer hungry. In this time of plenty, most of us on average carry enough fat reserves to get us through about a month!

Bottom line issues

Less going in means less coming out. It shouldn't require treatment unless you have mass bloating or abdominal discomfort. If this is the case, laxatives or magnesium supplements can be added. On the flip side, sometimes you may get a flush-out as your body clears toxins. Keep hydrated.

Headaches tend to disappear after the first few fasts. Taking some extra pink salt often helps (one-eighth of a teaspoon dissolved in water) and if your tummy gets the gurgles, mineral water may also help. Remain hydrated and supplement with sugar-free electrolytes.

If you truly don't feel well, get excessively dizzy, really weak or have other severe symptoms, then you should break your fast. Gently.

Top tips for fasting

- Hydrate—drink plenty water.
- Keep busy.
- Drink coffee or tea.
- Ride out the hunger.
- Give yourself time to see if daily intermittent fasting is a good fit for you. A month trial is a good period.
- Follow a lower-carb lifestyle between fasting. This reduces hunger and makes intermittent fasting much easier, because you're fat-adapted.
- Don't binge before or after fasting—go easy—eat nutrient dense, quality protein and fats.
- Break your fast gently. The longer the fast, the gentler you'll have to be.

Ketones

Another popular strategy is to introduce the natural bio-identical ketones I've spoken about previously. Ketones, as we have learned, burn your fat for fuel and are a signalling molecule. They are simply a most wonderful tool to extend fasting and minimise cravings. If you are considering adding ketones to help with insulin resistance, you can include them in fasting and they will not break your fast.

Bio identical and *natural* are the important words here. If you're going to consider using these as a tool, please make sure they are the naturally fermented ones and that they are the correct isomer. Quality ketones can cross the blood brain barrier, so they are also useful in reversing insulin resistance, especially in the brain. Not all exogenous (made externally) ketones are created equal. There are left-handed and right-handed ketones. There are some that fit the lock and some that jam it. Some are full of fillers, and some aren't. Don't make the mistake of taking ketones that aren't really ketones. I've added in some details about these in Appendix B for you because of some brands that 'fairy-dust' the active ingredients in miniscule amounts or utilise the incorrect isomer that jams the lock and can inadvertently sabotage your efforts. Please reach out to me for help with these.

Increase your salt intake

The risks associated with consuming too much salt have been vigorously debated for over a century, and most recently, salt has gone from something that was treasured, to something to be avoided. Authorities have been saying for decades to cut back on salt, especially for lowering blood pressure and heart disease risk, however sodium is an absolutely *essential* nutrient that *must* come from your diet because your body can't make it on its own.

> What you've been told, again, isn't accurate and evidence linking salt to heart disease is rubbery.

Your body uses salt to balance fluids and maintain a healthy blood pressure. Salt is *essential* for transmitting nerve impulses, assisting brain communication pathways and contracting and relaxing muscle fibres (including those in the heart and blood vessels)— therefore promoting muscle function. The human body can't live without some sodium. Your body will also stamp its feet, if you're low in this mineral, often with cramps, headaches and brain fog.

A recent study threatens to derail the whole anti-salt movement. A worldwide group of scientists collected over 100,000 adult urine samples from 17 countries. They observed their subjects' health over a period of four years. What they reported, was that consumption of *less* than four grams of sodium per day actually correlated with a s*harp increased risk* of death, almost *doubling*, when the subject reduced as low as two grams a day of sodium. What this means is that *no* sodium is more damaging to us than too much.

Another recent study by The American Journal of Hypertension involving 6,250 subjects, found *no strong evidence* that cutting salt intake reduced the risk for heart attacks, strokes or death in people with normal or high blood pressure in any way at all.

A 2006 American Journal of Medicine study compared daily sodium intake of almost 80 million Americans. to their risk of heart disease mortality over 14 years. It found that the *more* sodium people ate, the *less* likely they were to die from heart disease.

And yet more. A 2007 European Journal of Epidemiology study that followed 1,500 people for five years, *found no association* between urinary sodium levels and the risk of cardiovascular disease.

Hmm... tell me again why we are so very confused? All I can say is that with my doctor's supervision, I've been adding pink salt every day and my blood pressure has dropped, not risen. The blood test results I spoke about earlier, included tests on sodium levels and kidney function. All just fine. Being in ketosis accelerates sodium excretion by the kidneys, hence the need for supplementation. In contrast, a high-carbohydrate diet suppresses the kidneys' natural ability to excrete sodium and reduces your 'salt tolerance.' So, if you're lowering your carbs, salt will not kill you, it will only benefit you.

Bloating

When sodium is in short supply in the body, a host of hormonal messages tell the kidneys and sweat glands to hold onto the water in your system and conserve it. When you have more sodium than you need, your kidneys flush out the excess by making saltier urine. Alternatively, if they can't get rid of enough sodium, it accumulates in the fluid between cells. Water follows sodium—as the volume of this fluid increases, so does the volume of blood. This means more work for the heart and more pressure on blood vessels. When your body finally drops the water weight that is needed for glucose metabolism, it also takes with it a load of essential minerals, including sodium, magnesium and potassium. This should rectify over the first few weeks, but you may need to re-introduce these in order to combat 'keto-flu', which is really just de-mineralisation and dehydration.

For now, know that if you're cutting your carbs a little, upping your salt a little too is perfectly fine. With a diet rich in processed food, you were getting extra salt as an additive that you've cut out. When you lower processed food, it's vital you replace this salt intake.

A leading researcher in body metabolism, Dr Stephen Phinney says, *'In short, 3000–5000 mg of sodium and 3000–4000 mg of potassium on average are needed as part of a well-formulated ketogenic diet.'*

Consuming one-eighth of a teaspoon of pink salt dissolved in in water, either as a shot or in a glass, can help fire up your spark plugs again, kill the headaches, brain fog and give you back your zippiness.

Weather or not...

Know, too, as the weather in your region cools, you'll have the propensity to eat more, and be hunting for 'comfort foods' your body can store 'for the winter'. This is again, an ancestral hangover, from when food was scarce.

This primeval 'hunting' instinct can be counteracted by:

- cooking fatty cheaper meat cuts—low and slow.
- replacing starchy foods like potatoes and rice/pasta with loads of green veg and healthy fats.
- eating protein first, to get the stomach juices flowing.
- making some low carb treats or desserts, so you're not tempted to indulge (I have included loads of recipes in the back of the book for you).
- making water a priority, even in winter.

CHAPTER 13

Dances with brooms

'What we tell people to do to lose weight— eat less and exercise more—is exactly what you'd do if you wanted to make yourself hungry.'

GARY TAUBES

D id you know that the more you move, the hungrier you get? If weight loss was as simple as calories in, calories out and eat less move more, I'd be a supermodel by now.

Clearly, I'm not (yet).

The simple fact is that exercise alone *does not help with weight loss*- but that does *not* mean that exercising is not good for you, because it is. I am not saying you shouldn't exercise, because it's very healthy (unlike my relationship with exercise) for your mind, to build muscle mass and clean up your limbic system. However, exercise is of minor importance when it comes to weight loss. Is your mind blown yet?

In 1977, the US National Institutes of Health held a conference on weight control and obesity. They stated:

'The importance of exercise in weight control is less than might be believed, because increases in energy expenditure due to exercise also tend to increase food consumption and it is not possible to predict whether the increased caloric output will be outweighed by the greater food intake.'

Add movement—but not too much...

Did you know—by climbing 100 stairs you can burn 4.6 calories. Our friend, the donut, is worth 460 calories per 100 grams. That means to burn off ONE donut, you'd need to climb 1,000 stairs. One donut! And that is *before* you access the fat storage shed! Climbing stairs, however, is one of the best exercises when it comes to strength and toning—and paired with the immense good it does for your muscle mass, lungs and cardiovascular system, it's certainly worth doing, but *not* for the fat loss. I've got a great idea—you do the stairs; I'll go for a walk on the beach and get similar results. I know which I'd prefer, don't you?

A common approach for losing weight is to reduce calories and add more exercise. As this approach fails, most of us then lower our food intake even more and do even more exercise. This can cause us to become physically and mentally exhausted... with no real weight loss to show for our efforts. The longer you follow this approach, the more likely you are to overexercise and then overeat, which, in turn, adds an increasing amount of stress on our body. In the process, we speed up ageing and increase chronic inflammation. This approach is not sustainable, as you can probably attest to.

There was a time not so long ago when no one believed exercise would help with weight loss. Even until the 1960s, those who treated overweight patients dismissed the idea of exercise for weight loss as naive. Remember William Banting in our earlier chapters?

Exercise makes us hungry. Full stop. Burn more calories and the odds are pretty excellent that you'll consume more food as well.

When an obesity and diabetes specialist from the Mayo Clinic, Russell Wilder, spoke on obesity in 1932, he mentioned that his '*fat patients tended to lose more weight with bed rest; while unusually strenuous physical exercise slows the rate of loss.*'

It's your biology, not lack of willpower, that leads exercise to fail as a weight-loss tool. Because it is insulin and cortisol that determine fat accumulation, and we get fat not because we eat too much, or exercise too little, but because our body makes too much insulin, or our insulin levels remain elevated far longer than they were biologically meant to.

Gary Taubes, in an article for The Guardian, wrote:

'*Steve Blair, a University of South Carolina exercise scientist, says he was 'short, fat and bald' when he started running in his thirties and he is short, fatter and balder now, at age 68. In the intervening years, he estimates, he has run close to 80,000 miles and gained about 30lb.*' When Taubes asked Blair whether he thought he might be leaner had he run even more, he had to think about it. He said '*I don't see how I could have been more active. Thirty years ago, I was running 50 miles a week. I had no time to do more. But if I could have gone out over the last couple of decades for two to three hours a day, maybe I would not have gained this weight.'*

Hmmm.

Here's another one for you to consider. In 1989, a Danish study on physical activity and weight loss was published. Over 18 months, the Danes trained non-athletes to take part in a marathon. By the end of this period, 18 men in the study had lost an average of only two-and-a-half kilograms of body fat and the nine women had *'no change in body composition'*.

Please don't take this as a reason *not* to get active. A walk is amazing for your brain! You can live longer, perhaps even reduce your risk of heart disease or diabetes. You'll even feel better about yourself, as a twenty to thirty-minute walk improves general fitness, cardiac and brain health, boosts your mood, lowers stress and improves endurance, circulation and posture. It also improves your digestion, cleans up your limbic system and increases endorphins. Exercise also helps increase production of neurotransmitters that assist with quality sleep.

Twenty to thirty minutes, three to five times a week, can help maintain system health. You love me a lot now hey?

Health benefits of gentle/moderate exercise

- improved bone mineral density
- more robust immune system
- improves insulin sensitivity
- better brain health—exercise improves age-related cognitive decline and help prevent neurodegenerative diseases
- improved cardiovascular health and blood flow

If you're not a fan of working out (like me), find some alternatives to traditional exercise.

Expand your NEAT—Non-Exercise Activity Thermogenesis.

NEAT is energy expended for everything that isn't sleeping, eating or sports-like exercise. Energy used during walking, typing, gardening, playing with the kids, shopping, hanging the washing, sweeping the path, undertaking other home duties and even fidgeting—these are NEAT activities. Here's the cool thing—your metabolic rate can be substantially lifted by these seemingly trivial physical things.

Physiological studies have demonstrated that NEAT is increased with changes in energy; meaning you can do incidental movement, like mop the floors and upregulate your metabolism at the same time. Cool!

Some NEAT ideas include:

- garden—pull out some weeds, trim the hedges
- walk on the beach or go for a bushwalk
- listen to a podcast while you're walking
- dance with the broom to ABBA or join a class and wear leg warmers for the fun of it
- practise yoga or pilates
- walk the shopping centre
- park at the furthest end of the carpark and walk
- take the stairs instead of the lift or escalator
- strength/interval/resistance training is a great idea. (HIIT)
- include some rest days

Sleep

Sleep is a weapon that incinerates fat.

Research has shown if you don't get enough quality sleep, you'll be half as effective at losing fat, compared to those who get plenty of sleep. If that's not a reason to optimise your sleep, I don't know what is. Bed occupies a third of our life and is a physiological cyclical process that has an absolutely critical impact on our health and well-being. Sleep is integral for growth, learning, development, memory, emotion regulation, immune strengthening and, most importantly, cleaning out neuro-toxic substances from the brain.

Did you know that consecutive nights of poor sleep are actually as detrimental to your health as a poor diet?

Consistently great sleep also has been shown to decrease insulin resistance and cortisol, making it easier to maintain and lose weight. Sleep also holds sway over those two important appetite hormones in our body—leptin and ghrelin. If you're not sleeping well, your body creates more ghrelin to drive you to reach for fast energy. When we're tired, we might reach for a bag of jelly snakes, a coffee or energy drink. We might find the car making its way through the Macca's drive-through for a quick fix. Think about how you felt the last time you didn't get enough sleep. Did you feel a bit shabby and reach for something quick to eat with seemingly no will-power? We make worse food choices when we are tired because we simply need the energy.

In general, people who don't get enough sleep are also more prone to late-night snacking. The items that we reach for usually contain pretty large amounts of refined sugar and even worse, the lethal combo of glucose and seed oils. Yes, including Macca's *and* your favourite fast foods. These are quickly absorbed into our system and, if we don't burn them quickly, they turn straight into... you guessed it—fat. *Especially* at night, when it isn't burned.

Not getting enough sleep is also related to your body's ability to process insulin, leading to higher cortisol levels, compounding the effect.

Appetite aside, sleep is vitally important to a number of brain functions, including how nerve cells and neurons communicate with each other. Your brain stays highly active while you sleep.

One of the coolest discoveries in recent years, is that the brain removes accumulated toxins much more rapidly while you're asleep than when awake. While you are blissfully unaware, 'gunk' is cleared from your brain. Most of this is β-amyloid protein, which is linked to Alzheimer's affected brains. Researchers have learned that these proteins and toxins accumulate during the day and are cleared during sleep.

During sleep, your brain also cleans up the tens of thousands of new neural pathways it's made during the day. It arranges the filing cabinet so you can find stuff again. Sleep contributes to memory function by converting short-term learnings into long-term memories, as well as erasing unneeded information that might otherwise overload our system. Like performing a Marie Kondo clean-up on your home or a system defrag on your computer.

Sleep also seems to pin negative emotional memories. An interesting recent study shows that as negative experiences are consolidated in sleep, they are easier than other memories to access—this literally comes back to our brain wanting to protect us. It learns that 'bad memories' are things in day-to-day life to avoid—in case we should perish from this.

This is why starting your day by being grateful and getting enough sleep at the end is so *vitally* important. You can literally re-wire your brain with positivity and gratitude.

How to hack your sleep
- Create a sleep-friendly space—make sure your bed and pillow are comfortable. Make sure it's an ideal ambient temperature.
- Cut out light sources—this increases melatonin.
- Turn electronics off half an hour before bedtime.
- Avoid eating two to three hours before bed.
- Get into the open air and reset your circadian rhythm.
- Minimise alcohol and caffeine intake.
- Try not to nap during the day.
- Aim for consistency with sleep and wake times.

When you can't fall asleep
- Try box breathing. In for four, hold for four, out for four. Wait for four. Repeat. This calms your nervous system. You can also try counting ten in slowly, ten out slowly.
- Don't stew in bed—if your brain is busy, hop up and do something relaxing. Then try again. Stressing only induces cortisol and your body thinks you're going to be attacked by a predator.
- Several supplements can induce relaxation and help you sleep, including non-caffeinated ketones, ginkgo biloba, glycine, valerian root, magnesium, lavender.
- If all else fails, speak to your doctor.

Menopause madness

Sorry boys, this section is for the girls. For females, menopause can sabotage you too, as some of you well know. Bloody hormones. At the start of menopause, a woman's rate of fat-gain *doubles* and lean muscle mass declines. This is due to hormonal changes and not simply age—and it continues approximately two years after the final menstrual period before it stabilises. Symptoms of menopause are hormonal and include hot flashes and night sweats, mood changes and brain fog, headaches, disrupted sleep, bloating and, unfortunately, increased abdominal body fat. Most women, (without any change in diet or lifestyle), gain an average of one to three kilograms during menopausal transition. Since I've been following this lifestyle, my menopause symptoms have all but disappeared, which is very exciting!

Also, during menopause, a significant increase in secretion of cortisol is likely, especially during sleep. Yay! Not. This is why its vitally important to lower insulin and cortisol as a menopausal female as much as you can, and restore hormone balance.

Eight tips for minimising menopause symptoms:
- Lower your carb intake—this keeps insulin low and maintains metabolism.
- Consume adequate protein—this helps maintain lean muscle mass.
- Lift light weights or do some resistance training. This also helps maintain muscle—important as you age to protect against 'having a fall'.
- Introduce fasting, or time-restricted eating keeping insulin low for longer stretches.
- Avoid over-consumption of snacks, nuts and alcohol, particularly late at night.

- Make sleep a priority.
- Manage stress with yoga, breathing, light exercise, playing with kids, reading, walking or gardening.
- Try natural exogenous ketones, that help with sleep, energy, mood and cravings.
- Talk to your doctor about a trial of hormone replacement therapy (HRT) if you are having a very difficult menopause transition.

Understanding alcohol

Warning—you may not love me so much after reading this next bit. One of the biggest saboteurs on your journey is alcohol. If you're experiencing a plateau, leave the alcohol in the bottle. It can slow or even halt weight loss because our body *has* to prioritise alcohol—it cannot store it. Technically, it's a toxin.

The reason your nightly wine slows weight loss, is not because of its calories, but because it impedes the body's ability to utilise fat stores for energy. Unlike glucose, fructose and alcohol go straight to the liver, where they are metabolised in almost exactly the same way. When consumed in excess, both can promote fatty liver, leading to eventual liver fibrosis, scarring and potentially cirrhosis —liver damage where healthy cells are replaced by scar tissue, liver failure and even liver cancer. Definitely not as cheerful, as a weekend cheers with friends.

Once ingested, alcohol must be burnt immediately. It *must* take precedence over any foods we consume or even what we have eaten previously that day. When alcohol is consumed, it's broken down into acetate, which is burned before any other stored energy and the body will give preferential treatment to acetate over sugar and fat. In other words, your body will cling to the treats you had earlier in the day or week and prioritise the alcohol. The surplus gets turned into... fat. That bloody F-word again. That's why plateaus are so common for people who enjoy alcohol but have goals of fat loss.

You've heard alcohol kills brain cells, but alcohol doesn't actually kill them. It damages the ends of the neurons, (dendrites) which makes it difficult for them to transmit messages to one another. Heavy and binge drinking can result in permanent damage to the brain, causing chronic changes in brain pathways.

Alcohol is also a well-known appetite booster. We are less able to fend off cravings for chips, sweets and other rich foods if we've had a few. A drink or three makes these snacks go down the hatch faster than you can say 'Alice in Wonderland'. As our inhibitions fall to the wayside, with each drink, we find ourselves eating more than our share of the grazing table or hoeing into ice cream, snacks or treats that we'd normally have the willpower to resist or just have a handful off, rather than a bucketful.

If you're looking to gain weight, scientifically the best approach is to drink a lot of alcohol and eat chips at the same time.

You don't have to give up alcohol completely, in order to lose or maintain your fat stores. However, it certainly will help. Many alcoholic beverages are also very high in sugars, with some having over 30 grams in a *single* serving. This is five times what your body is designed to handle. Cocktails and mixed drinks also rely on high-carb, sugary ingredients like fruit juice, mixers, sweeteners or syrups. Even regular beer is produced from grain and can host 12 grams of carbs or more in a can.

Here are some alternatives if you're trying to minimise insulin and reduce fat storage (grams (g) = sugar content)

Avoid		Better choices	
Margarita	1 cup = 13g	Rum	44 ml 0g
Bloody Mary	1 cup = 10g	Vodka	44 m 0g
Whiskey sour	1 nip =14g	Gin	44 ml 0g
Sangria	1 cup = 20g	Tequila	44 ml 0g
Piña colada	½ cup = 32g	Whiskey	44 ml 0g
Cosmopolitan	⅓ cup = 22g	Red wine	½ glass 3–4g
Regular beer	355 ml can = 12 grams	White wine	½ glass 3–4g
		Sweet wine	½ glass 8–10g
		Light beer	355 ml 3g

Hack

You may like to add a sparkle to these with soda water, unsweetened tonic water or mineral water, to make a satisfying thirst quencher or blood sugar friendlier cocktail.

Tips for reducing alcohol consumption

- Know your priorities—understand it will sabotage your health and waistline.
- Drink water first.
- Measure your drinks and stick to your agreed limit.
- Offer to be the designated driver in social situations.
- Space out your drinks and drink water between.
- Add ice or sparkling water to your drink.
- Go for a walk if the cravings are calling.
- Look for lower-carb choices.
- Eat good clean food before alcohol consumption.
- Prepare keto friendly snacks beforehand.

CHAPTER 14

There is no wagon

W hy do we all want such quick results when it took us so long to get here in the first place? If you truly want to be metabolically flexible, without ever following another diet, you must give it time and be gentle on yourself. This is *not* a race. *It's your life.*

You are not a tree. You can decide to move, flourish, or change the trajectory of your life with just one decision, *even* if that decision is remade every day. Instead of riding the, '*Oh fuck, I fell off, I'm beating myself up,*' roundabout, you can *decide* to make a choice and leave the oops blip in your past. Step on over it.

There is no such thing as failing, only learning.

What tripped you over? Was it the chips that fell in your mouth, or the block of chocolate you ate while watching *Big Brother*? Are you *really* going to let that *one* slip, that *one* teeny, tiny, insignificant, momentary event determine your health for the *rest of your life?* Heck, no! If you consider this a lifestyle of learnings, you can jump back on any time you damn well want to.

Decide to get back on, no matter what.

Have a think about how long it took you to get here and the path you've already walked. I shared my stories with you, in the hope you can relate and recognise some of the events in your life that have led you to *right now.* How long, realistically, are you expecting it to take to undo the events and previous damage of your past?

You are not a tree.

If you *truly* want to be free from walking into a room and wondering what on earth you went there for, senior and blonde moments, long term permanent brain deterioration and the craving merry-go-round, then *all* you need to do is make a *conscious decision* to do this for *you*—and for your brain. Know that you can move forward at any time—and *choose* to move forward with freedom, without the guilt, without the sense of failure. *There is no better time.*

The time is *now.*

Getting up from tripping over.

- Make a choice—a choice to simply minimise blood sugar.
- Reset. Retake measurements and photos. This sends a message to your brain that it is really happening.
- If you fall off—get back on—know it's only a stumble, not a failure.

- Push out your eating window by a few more hours. Try a longer fast to kick your fat burning into gear.
- Tap into a community—look for low carb meet-ups and workshops in your area.
- Track your macros for a week—there are loads of great tracking apps. Make sure you're not over or under eating.
- Try natural bio-identical ketones. The real stuff, not the pretenders.
- Allow your body the time and grace to detox.
- Be aware of sneaky grains and hidden sugar.
- Remove processed food that may have crept in (or hasn't left).
- Listen to some inspirational podcasts.
- Get educated with books and resources—I've listed some in a few pages for you.
- Check out coaching courses or work with someone who understands this lifestyle, someone who has walked this road before you (I can help you).
- Forgive yourself, let go of the guilt—and understand that this will take time. Guilt is *more damaging* than the actual slip-up.

And finally, be gentle and kind to *you*. Reward yourself for little achievements and learn from your mistakes. Little by little, you can unlock some answers, and more importantly, results.

You didn't get here overnight, so give this time and know that wagons are for falling off and then, most importantly, getting back on.

Afterward

A nd you've made it. The rest is up to you. I believe you can do this. I know, because I've been there. Know without any shadow of a doubt, that this is a lifestyle, not a diet. Know that you get better at it, and it's one where you're *allowed* to make mistakes, as long as you learn from them. Nobody will die from eating one bag of chips. However, you, your brain, and your health won't be optimised if the single bag turns into 10. Re-read any chapter you need to, and know that if you don't start today, you'll be *exactly* where you were before you started.

Because you've made it this far—I'd like to gift you a free mini-tutorial. Check out my free video tutorial: *Simple Changes for Extraordinary Results* tinyurl. com/thefwordtipswebinar for the easiest way to begin.

Some of my most successful customers have joined and completed one of my personally coached courses, where I share with you, all my secret simple strategies for permanently losing the squish, regaining your brain and never having to follow another diet. *Ever...* You can find more of this information in Appendix B.

What if you *just began?*

In a year's time, please don't be sitting here, without having made a commitment to yourself, because if you don't make some of the little changes I've suggested, that is *exactly* where you'll be. Start today.

I'd love to offer you a hand if you need it. Please send me your commitment and goals—email me at: thefwordmatters@gmail.com and I'll send you a personalised message of support. I believe in you, and now, it's *your turn.*

Hugs, Emma xx

Inspiring information

Podcasts

- *Low-Carb MD*
- *Low-Carb Down Under*—Dr Paul Mason
- Dr Eric Berg
- *The Obesity Code*—Dr Jason Fung

Educational websites

- Virtahealth.com
- The Charlie Foundation
- Diet doctor.com
- The Fasting Lane website
- The Keto Life Group on Facebook
- Pruvit.tv

Inspiring people

- Peter Attia—mindset
- BU by Brian Underwood—mindset
- Robb Wolfe – author of Wired to Eat
- Benjamin Bikman PhD – science and research
- Tom Bilyeu—keto proof and science
- Joe Rogan—keto proof and motivation
- Dr Domonique D'Agostino—science and research
- Dr Lillianne Mujica-Parodi—science and research
- Dr Daniel Amen—brain research
- Dr Eric Berg—great quick tips
- Dr John Yudkin—sugar
- Dr Paul Mason—*Low-Carb Down Under* podcast
- Dr David Diamond—research on cholesterol and statins
- Dr Eric Westman
- Dr Jeff Volek

Books

- *Big Fat Lies*—David Gillespie
- *Sweet Poison*—David Gillespie
- *Fat Chance* –Robert Lustig
- *Good Calories, Bad Calories*—Gary Taubes
- *The Big Fat Surprise*—Nina Teicholz
- *Why We Get Fat*—Gary Taubes
- *The Case Against Sugar*—Gary Taubes
- *Grain Brain*—Dr David Perlmutter
- *The Obesity Code*—Dr Jason Fung
- *The Fasting Lane*—Dr Jason Fung, Eve Mayer and Megan Ramos
- *Why We Get Sick*—Benjamin Bikman, PhD

- *The Art and Science of Low-Carbohydrate Living*—Dr Stephen Phinney
- *The Art and Science of Low-Carbohydrate Performance*—Jeff Volek and Stephen Phinney
- *Wired to Eat*—Robb Wolf
- *Fat Chance*—Dr Robert Lustig
- *Metabolic*—Dr Robert Lustig
- *Keto Clarity: Your Definitive Guide to the Benefits of a Low-Carb, High-Fat Lifestyle*—Jimmy Moore and Eric C. Westman, M.D
- *New Atkins for a New You*—Eric Westman, Stephen Phinney, Jeff Volek
- *Life Without Bread*—Christian B. Allan and Wolfgang Lutz
- *The Real Meal Revolution*—Tim Noakes, Jonno Proudfoot, Sally-Ann Creed
- *Low-Carb, High-Fat Food Revolution: Advice and Recipes to Improve Your Health and Reduce Your Weight*—By: Andreas Eenfeldt

Documentaries

- *Fat: A Documentary*
- *The Magic Pill*
- *Cereal Killers*
- *The Truth about Sugar*—BBC
- *Fathead*
- *Sugar Rush*—Jamie Oliver
- *That Sugar Film*
- *The Sugar Conspiracy*
- *Fat Fiction*
- *Carb Loaded*
- *Fed Up*
- *Food Inc*

- *What's with Wheat*
- *Fat Fiction*
- *My Big Fat Diet*
- *Sugar Coated*
- *Sugar—The Bitter Truth*
- *Toxic Sugar*
- *Foods That Make Billions*—BBC Documentary
- *Fast Food Baby*—– BBC Documentary
- *The Big Fat Surprise*—Nin Teicholz
- *The Straight Dope on Cholesterol*—Peter Attia
- *The Secrets of Sugar—The Fifth Estate*—CBC
- *King Corn*
- *Sugar Crash*
- *The Skinny on Fat* series
- *Tim Noakes on trial*

The recipe files

When food is easy, this lifestyle is a no-brainer. If there's something you want that isn't included here, just search for it in Google and add 'keto' or 'low-carb' in front. There are many resources on the internet, which is where I found most of these and adapted them. I've personally made each of these recipes and they are the best-loved of all.

These simple recipes, that are blood sugar-friendly and satisfying won't spike your fat storage response. These assisted me to replace foods I was initially craving. I've got masses more family friendly recipes in saveable photos—head on over to my private Facebook group, The Lazy Keto Mum: https://tinyurl.com/lazyketomumgroup—at last count, there are 330+ recipes, all of which you can save straight to your device. You'll find a lovely supportive community there too.

You can also follow me as I share new tips and recipes:
www.facebook.com/TheLazyKetoMum and
https://tinyurl.com/emmamtiktok

Keto pantry staples

(Also see shopping list – Appendix A)

Dry Flours

Almond flour
Coconut flour
Chia flour
Psyllium husk

Friendly Sweeteners

Powdered Erythritol
Liquid stevia
Monkfruit

Baking and Cooking Aids

Keto baking flour–1:2 ratio of bicarbonate and cream of tartar
Cream of tartar
Bicarbonate of soda
Xanthan gum
Vanilla
Vinegars (no sugar)
Tamari (wheat-free soy)
Salt and pepper

Oil

Olive oil
Coconut oil
Avocado oil
Drippings collected from meat
Coconut milk and cream

Refrigerated Items

Butter
Ghee
Almond or coconut milk
Eggs
Cream
Meats
Green vegetables

SIMPLE SNACKS

KETO DIP

Ingredients
200 g block of full fat cream cheese
2 tsp olive oil
30 g fresh chopped parsley or fresh basil
1 garlic clove, minced
1 tsp lemon zest
salt and pepper, to taste

Method
Stir all ingredients into the softened cream cheese. Refrigerate for at least 10 minutes to let all the flavours develop. Add salt if needed. Feel free to experiment with other herbs and spices. Serve with the crackers on the next few pages.

SOUR CREAM AND CHIVE CRACKERS

Ingredients
2 cups almond flour
Small bunch (20 g) fresh chives
70 g full-fat sour cream
$\frac{1}{2}$ tsp garlic powder
1 tsp Himalayan salt

Method
Preheat the oven to 100 °C. Chop the chives into small pieces.

In a medium bowl, mix all the ingredients by hand. Knead for a half a minute or until smooth. Place the dough on a baking tray lined with baking paper. Place another sheet of baking paper on the dough. Using a rolling pin, roll the dough between the two baking papers as thinly as possible. Remove the topmost baking paper.

Cut the dough with a knife or pizza cutter into squares.

Place in oven and bake for 50–60 minutes. Check frequently so that the crackers don't get too dark or burnt.

Cool completely and break into squares. You can also use this as a marvellous quiche base!

KETO CRACKERS

Ingredients
180 g sesame seeds
70 g sunflower seeds
60 g shredded cheddar cheese (omit if dairy free)
1 tbsp ground psyllium husk
120 ml water
2 eggs
$\frac{1}{4}$ tsp salt
salt and pepper, to taste

Method
Preheat the oven to 180°C. Line a 30 x 40 baking tray with baking paper. Add all the ingredients to a medium bowl and stir until combined. Spread the mix a few mm thick onto the paper, sprinkle with salt and bake for approximately 20 minutes. Remove from the oven, carefully cut into preferred shape.

Lower the heat to 140°C and pop back into oven for another 30–40 minutes, or until lightly golden in colour.

Check the crispbread to make sure it is completely dry. Keep it in the oven with the door slightly open and cool in the oven.

KETO PARMESAN CRACKERS

Ingredients
1 cup grated parmesan cheese
½ tsp linseeds
½ tsp poppy seeds
½ tsp chia seeds
1 tsp sesame seeds
¼ tsp pink salt

Method
Preheat the oven to 180°C. Line a 30 x 40 baking tray with a silicone baking matt. Place 1 tsp—1 tbsp (amount influences the size of the cracker) in little piles on your tray approximately 1 inch apart and flatten—the thinner they are the crispier they will be. Allow room for spreading. In a small bowl, combine seeds and salt. Sprinkle over flattened cheese and bake for approximately 20 minutes or until golden. Allow to cool before eating.

DEVILLED EGGS

Ingredients
6 large eggs, hard boiled
¼ cup sugar free mayonnaise (recipe in sauces section)
1 tbsp Dijon mustard
salt and pepper to taste

Optional garnishes
paprika
spring onion
sesame seeds

Method
Hard boil eggs and peel. Slice in half lengthwise.

Remove the yolks and mix them in a bowl with mayo, mustard, salt and pepper. Spoon the filling into each egg white and finish with garnishes.

MINI EGG FRITTATAS—THREE WAYS

Ingredients
BASE:
12 large eggs
2 tbsp very finely chopped onion
salt and pepper, to taste

TOMATO SPINACH MOZZARELLA:
¼ cup fresh spinach, roughly chopped
8 cherry tomatoes, halved
¼ cup shredded mozzarella cheese

BACON CHEDDAR:
¼ cup cooked bacon, chopped
¼ cup shredded cheddar cheese

GARLIC MUSHROOM PEPPER:
¼ cup sliced brown mushrooms
¼ cup red bell pepper (capsicum), diced
1 tbsp fresh chopped parsley
¼ tsp garlic powder or ⅓ teaspoon minced garlic

Method

Preheat oven to 180°C. Lightly spray a 12-cup muffin tin with coconut oil spray. In a large bowl, whisk eggs and onion. Season with salt and pepper, to taste. Add egg mixture halfway up into each tin area. Divide the three topping combos equally.

Bake for 15—20 minutes, until set. Let cool slightly, then serve or store in an airtight container in the fridge for up to 4 days and reheat when ready to serve or eat cold.

You can really add any filling to these—try experimenting with adding leftover finely chopped roast or other vegetables.

KETO MUG CAKE

Ingredients

2 tbsp almond flour

1 tbsp cocoa powder

2 tbsp powdered erythritol

$\frac{1}{2}$ tsp baking powder

4 tsp vanilla extract

1 pinch salt

1 egg, beaten

1 $\frac{1}{2}$ tbsp melted coconut oil or butter

$\frac{1}{2}$ tsp coconut oil or butter for greasing the mug

$\frac{1}{2}$ tbsp coarsely chopped sugar-free dark chocolate (I like Lindt 85-90% plus cocoa solids)

Method

Combine dry ingredients in a small bowl. Add eggs, melted coconut oil/butter and chocolate. Mix until smooth.

Equally divide batter into 2 well-greased coffee mugs or microwave-safe ramekins (⅔ filled).

Microwave method: Microwave on high for 1–1 ½ minutes (700 watts). Remove and allow to cool for 1 minute.

Oven method: Preheat your oven to 180°C.

Instead of a mug, place liners in a muffin pan and fill them halfway.

Bake for about 12–14 minutes or springy to the touch when pressing gently in the middle. Cool.

OVEN BAKED CHEESE

Ingredients
260 g brie or camembert cheese
1 garlic clove, minced
1 tbsp fresh rosemary, coarsely chopped
55 g pecans or walnuts, coarsely chopped
1 tbsp olive oil
salt and pepper

Method
Preheat the oven to 200°C. Place the cheese on a baking tray lined with baking paper or in a small non-stick baking dish.

In a little bowl, mix garlic, herbs and nuts together with olive oil. Add salt and pepper to taste. Place the nut mixture on the cheese and bake for 10 minutes or until cheese is warm and soft and nuts are toasted. Serve warm or lukewarm. You're welcome!

KETO HOT CHOC

Ingredients
30 g unsalted butter
1 tbsp cacao powder
2½ tsp powdered erythritol
¼ tsp vanilla extract
240 ml boiling water

Method
Put the ingredients in a tall cup to use with a liquid safe blender.

Mix for 15–20 seconds or until there's a fine foam on top.

Pour the hot cocoa carefully into to cups and enjoy. Add a glug of cream if you can tolerate dairy.

KETO FRENCH TOAST

Ingredients
MUG BREAD
1 tsp butter
2 tbsp almond flour
2 tbsp coconut flour
1 ½ tsp baking powder
1 pinch salt
2 eggs
2 tbsp heavy cream

BATTER
2 eggs
2 tbsp heavy whipping cream
½ tsp ground cinnamon
1 pinch salt
2 tbsp butter

Method
Grease a large mug or dish with a flat bottom with butter.

Mix together dry ingredients in the mug with a fork or spoon. Crack in the egg and stir in cream. Combine until smooth—make sure it's not lumpy. Microwave on high (approximately 700 watts) for 2 minutes. Check if the bread is set in the middle—if not, microwave for another 15–30 seconds. Let cool and remove from the mug. Slice in half.

In a bowl or deep plate, whisk together the eggs, cream and cinnamon with a pinch of salt. Pour over the bread slices and let them get soaked. Turn them around a few times so the bread slices absorb as much of the egg mixture as possible.

Fry in plenty of butter and serve immediately.

KRISPY CHICKEN SKINS

Ingredients
250 g chicken skin
½ tsp paprika powder
½ tsp garlic powder
½ tsp salt
¼ tsp ground black pepper

Method

Preheat oven to 200°C. Place chicken skin pieces on a baking tray and sprinkle with the seasoning. Bake in the oven for 15 minutes or until crispy.

MAKE A KETO TASTER PLATE!

Great inclusions:

cheese

olives

salmon

nuts

nitrate free meats and salami

almonds and pecans

keto dip

sliced green dippers like cucumber and celery

keto crackers

cauliflower florets

boiled eggs

beef jerky

baby tomatoes

smoked salmon

SIMPLE SWEETS

EMMA'S EASY NO BAKE CHEESECAKE
(YES, IT'S THE ONE FROM THE COVER!)

Ingredients
BASE
2 tbsp butter, melted
200 g almond flour
pinch of salt
1 tbsp powdered erythritol

Cheesecake
1 cup thickened cream
500 g cream cheese
150 g sour cream
3–4 tbsp powdered erythritol—to taste
¼ cup finely ground chia seeds (white is best)
1 tsp vanilla essence

Method
Blitz your chia seeds as finely as you can in a blender. Set aside.

BASE
Mix melted butter into almond flour, powdered erythritol and salt and press into a greased springform pan. I put baking paper on the bottom too. It makes it easier to serve. Refrigerate for at least 30 minutes.

CHEESECAKE
Beat cream to stiff peaks. Beat in softened cream cheese and then sour cream. Add erythritol, chia flour and vanilla and beat till smooth. Add more erythritol to taste if needed.

206

At this point you can quickly mix in any flavourings like lemon zest, orange zest, keto caramel, berries, cocoa or a combo like mocha—coffee and chocolate. Dollop over cold base and refrigerate till set.

If you like, you can drizzle it with any of these options below too.

KETO JAM

This can be drizzled over the top of the cheesecake once set, or ⅓ cup mixed into the cream cheese mix before spooning on the base.

Ingredients
700 g frozen or fresh berries
1 tsp lemon or lime zest
juice of a small lemon plus pips (put the pips in a muslin cloth for easy removal)
A few drops of liquid stevia
2–3 tbsp powdered erythritol

Method
Heat berries in a medium size pan on medium heat. Add the rest of the ingredients. Bring to the boil and cook further for approximately 30 minutes, until roughly half of the volume remains. Stir frequently. Taste and add more sweetener as desired—berries are all different and require different levels of sweetness. Start with a little—add more if needed. Remove from heat and take out the pips. Store in the fridge once cool.

KETO CARAMEL SAUCE
This can be mixed into the cheesecake too—
just ⅓ cup at the end before spooning onto base.
Drizzle the rest over the cheesecake.

Ingredients
½ cup cream
2 tbsp butter
2 tsp powdered erythritol

Method
Melt butter in a small pan. Simmer till brown—don't let it burn. Add cream and sweetener and cook till the sauce thickens— approximately 15 minutes. Allow to cool.

KETO COOKIE DOUGH BALLS

Ingredients
½ cup softened butter
⅓ cup powdered erythritol or 1 pack Kreme
1 tsp vanilla
½ tsp pink salt
2 cups almond flour/meal
½ cup 85–90% dark chocolate rough chopped into ½ cm sized chips

Method
Beat butter till fluffy and smooth. Add in sweetener. Mix in vanilla and salt. Add almond flour. You may need to add a little more depending on the almond flour consistency. Add chopped chocolate and roll into balls. Refrigerate. I make big batches and keep a mix frozen ready to make more at a moment's notice. You can also add a few drops of food grade orange or peppermint oil into these for a twist.

KETO BROWNIES

Ingredients
100 g 90% dark chocolate
½ cup butter
3 eggs
1 cup powdered (I love brown) erythritol
⅔ cup almond flour/meal
¼ cup cacao powder
¼ tsp pink salt
½ tsp xanthan gum
1 tsp granulated coffee
1 tsp baking powder

Method
Preheat oven to 180°C.
Prepare and grease a 20 x 20cm baking tray.
Break chocolate into pieces and melt with butter in a saucepan or microwave safe jug. Allow to cool slightly.
Whisk eggs in a separate bowl with powdered erythritol.
Mix remaining dry ingredients in large bowl. Slowly fold in egg mixture until combined.
Then add in butter and chocolate mixture. Don't beat! Be gentle but combine well.
You can also add keto friendly nuts at this point.
Pour into prepared baking tray and bake for 20 minutes.
Allow to cool in the tray. Enjoy by itself or with whipped cream and berries.

LOW-CARB FUDGE

Ingredients
1 cup cream
60 g dark chocolate (85–90% minimum cocoa solids)
150 g almond butter
3–4 tsp powdered erythritol
1–2 tsp vanilla

Method
Line a tray or container with baking paper. Mix almond butter and cream—set aside. In a glass bowl melt chocolate slowly. Either microwave or over steaming water. Add sweetener and vanilla. Mix in cream mixture. Pour into prepared tray. Allow to cool in freezer. Once frozen, it will keep for ages. Allow to soften before eating. Cut while frozen.

KETO CHOCOLATE

Ingredients
$\frac{1}{2}$ cup coconut oil
$\frac{1}{2}$ cup coconut butter
$\frac{1}{2}$ cup cacao
$\frac{1}{4}$ cup powdered erythritol
1 cup shredded coconut (optional)
Pinch of salt

Method
Slowly melt oil and butter on very low heat, add the other ingredients and mix well. Spread onto tray with baking paper, or chocolate moulds—into the freezer. Great for easter time (or late night oops).

KETO CHOC MOUSSE

Ingredients

300 ml thickened cream.

¼ cup cacao

2–3 tbsp powdered erythritol

Sprinkle of cinnamon and nutmeg (optional)

Beat till soft peaks form. Add in cacao and erythritol and mix well. Add a little—then more if needed. Serve with berries and mint. A crowd pleaser. Sometimes my daughter has this for breakfast.

KETO CHIA PUDDINGS

Ingredients

2 tbsp chia seeds

1 cup nut or coconut milk

1 tbsp powdered erythritol

Method

Mix chia seeds with milk and sweetener and stir to combine. Allow to chill, stirring occasionally. Overnight is best or at least a few hours. Top with cream, berries and the sugar free jam for a real treat. I topped mine with flaked almonds too.

GOOEY FUDGE BROWNIES
(not keto but low-sugar)

Ingredients
200 g dark, dairy-free chocolate (Lindt 85–90% works well)
130 g raw Medjool dates, pitted
180 g coconut oil
30 g coconut flour
4 eggs
½ tsp vanilla extract
¼ tsp sea salt

Instructions—this is for a Thermomix.
Preheat oven to 190°C. Line a 22cm square baking dish with baking paper. Place the chocolate (broken into pieces) into the mixing bowl and mill for 10 seconds on speed 9. Add the dates to the bowl and chop for 15 seconds on speed 10. Add the coconut oil and cook for 5 minutes at 60°C on speed 2.

Add remaining ingredients and mix for 20 seconds on speed 8. Scrape down lid and sides of bowl and mix for another 10 seconds on speed 6.

Scrape mixture into a lined, square baking dish. Bake in preheated 190°C oven for 18–20 minutes. Be careful not to overcook or they won't be gooey! Just until a skewer inserted in the centre comes out clean.

Cool then cut into small squares and refrigerate until cold.

EASY DINNERS

KETO FATHEAD PIZZA

CRUST
170 g mozzarella cheese, shredded
2 tbs cream cheese
85 g almond flour
1 tsp vinegar
1 egg
½ tsp salt
olive oil, to grease your hands

TOPPING
230 g fresh Italian sausage
1 tbs butter
120 ml unsweetened tomato sauce
½ tsp dried oregano
170 g mozzarella cheese, shredded

Method
Preheat the oven to 200°C.

Heat mozzarella and cream cheese in a non-stick pan on medium heat or in a bowl in the microwave oven.

Stir until they melt together. Add other ingredients and mix well.

Moisten your hands with olive oil and flatten the dough on baking paper, making a circle about 20cm round. You can also use a rolling pin to flatten the dough between two sheets of baking paper.

Remove the top sheet (if used).

Prick the crust with a fork (all over) and bake for 10–15 minutes until golden brown.

Flip the base and let it brown on the other side. Remove from the oven and cool. While the crust is cooling, lightly toast the ground sausage meat in olive oil or butter. Spread a thin layer of tomato sauce on the crust. Top the pizza with meat and plenty of cheese. Bake again for 10—15 minutes or until the cheese has melted. Sprinkle with oregano and enjoy!

This fathead dough can really form the basis for most bread recipes. Add any toppings your heart desires.

LOW-CARB QUICHE

Ingredients
1 quantity sour cream cracker dough mix
4 slices of bacon, diced
½ brown onion, diced
½ cup cheese, grated
3 eggs
1 ½ cups whipping cream
1 tsp Dijon mustard
1 pinch pink salt
2 pinches white pepper

Method
Sauté the diced bacon and onion in a non-stick frying pan over medium heat until the onion is translucent.

Spread the bacon and onion mixture evenly over the cooked base and top with the grated cheese.

In a small bowl, place the eggs, cream, mustard, salt and pepper, blend or whisk, ensuring that all ingredients are well combined.

Gently pour the cream mixture over the bacon, onion and cheese

Place the quiche back in the oven and bake for 25–35 minutes, the quiche is ready when the centre no longer jiggles when moved.

Remove from the oven. Cool slightly before serving.

KETO BIG MAC SALAD

Ingredients
500 g mince
1 tsp pink salt
¼ tsp pepper
1—2 cups shredded lettuce
1 cup tomatoes (chopped)
¾ cup cheddar cheese (shredded)
½ cup diced pickles or gherkins

Dressing
½ cup sugar free mayonnaise
2 tbsp pickles/gherkins, diced
2 tsp mustard
1 tsp vinegar
½ tsp paprika

Method
Cook mince in a pan over high heat. Season with salt and pepper. Brown the mince, breaking up the pieces, for about 7–10 minutes, until moisture has evaporated.

Meanwhile, combine all the dressing ingredients in a small bowl. If dressing is thicker than you like, thin out with water or oil. Refrigerate until ready to serve.

Combine the remaining salad ingredients in a large bowl. Add the meat mixture. Drizzle with dressing.

KETO CAULIFLOWER POTATO SALAD

Ingredients
500 g cauliflower
⅓ cup mayonnaise
1 tbsp olive oil
2 tbsp white vinegar
1 tbsp Dijon mustard
1 tsp garlic powder
¼ tsp paprika
½ tsp celery or pink salt
¼ tsp pepper
2 eggs hard boiled, chopped
¼ cup red onion sliced
¼ cup spring onions chopped

Instructions
Steam the cauliflower until fork tender, about 10 minutes. Cool to room temperature for 20–30 minutes.

Whisk the next 8 ingredients together, taste and adjust salt if needed. Stir the dressing in the bowl with the cauliflower then add in the onion, eggs and spring onions. Chill for 30 minutes or until ready to serve. Diced and toasted bacon is yum in this too.

SIMPLE KETO SALAD

chicken
bacon
avocado
spinach, kale or lettuce and green leaves of any type
Keto dressing—as much as you like—see below for recipes.

LOW-CARB CAULIFLOWER RICE

Ingredients
½ head cauliflower
2 tbsp butter
½ tsp salt

Method
Cut the cauliflower into evenly sized florets and place into your food processor, only filling half the bowl at a time.

Blend the cauliflower using the pulse setting. Continue to pulse until it resembles rice. If there are any large pieces, remove them and blend them separately. Heat a frying pan over medium heat. Add the butter and salt, allow the butter to melt before adding the cauliflower. Sauté the cauliflower for 5–8 minutes, whilst continually stirring. Remove from heat and serve. You can also make fried rice from this by adding other ingredients such as bacon, leek, slivers of carrot, little broccoli florets, etc.

KETO CURRY CHICKEN

Ingredients

1 small onion, roughly chopped

1 large green chili, roughly chopped (optional)

1-inch ginger, roughly chopped

3 cloves garlic

½ cup coriander, leaves and stalks

3 tbsp ghee or butter

2 tsp ground turmeric

1 ½ tsp ground cumin

1 tsp ground coriander

2 tbsp tomato paste

1 kg de-boned chicken thighs

1 cup full fat cream (or full fat yogurt)

1 tsp salt

Method

In your food processor, add the onion, green chili, ginger, garlic and fresh coriander. Blend until all ingredients are finely chopped. If your food processor is struggling, add a tablespoon of oil or water to help the ingredients move around. Scrape into a large saucepan over low heat, add the ghee and gently sauté for 10 minutes until fragrant.

Add the turmeric, cumin and ground coriander and continue to gently sauté for another 5 minutes. Add tomato paste and stir well to combine with the other ingredients, continue to cook for another 2 minutes before adding the diced chicken.

Increase the heat to medium and cook the chicken in the spices for 10 minutes. Add the cream and salt and reduce the heat until the curry is simmering. Simmer for 20–25 minutes until the chicken is cooked and sauce thickened.

MY GRANDMA'S SLOW COOKED LAMB

This is one of the best roast lamb recipes you'll ever find, I cook it when I'm time poor.

Ingredients
1 shoulder lamb
1 carrot
2–3 sticks celery
1 onion
2 garlic cloves
1 cup water and a stock cube
Few sprigs rosemary

Method
Preheat oven to 150°C. In a deep baking tray brown the lamb shoulder on the stovetop. Brown the roughly diced vegetables. Add the garlic at the end or else it burns.) Add a cup or two of water (enough to make a 1 cm layer over the base of the pan) and bring to the boil. Add the stock cube over the lamb. Season with salt and pepper.

Carefully take off the stovetop and cover in alfoil. Place in the oven for 5–6 hours. Watch your meat fall off the bone! Make a gravy with the pan juices, using a little corn-starch mixed in 1 tbsp water to thicken the gravy—this is not technically keto, but gravy is imperative. A keto friendly option is a little xanthan gum.

SLOW COOKED PORK BELLY
(another fave in our family)

Ingredients
1 piece pork belly
2–3 sticks celery, cut into chunks
2–3 onions
2 garlic cloves
1 cup water and a chicken stock cube
Salt

Method
Preheat oven to 150°C. Pat dry the top of your pork and make diagonal crosses in the skin from one side to the other. Both directions so you have diamond patterns—be careful not to cut the meat. Rub the skin with some oil and salt. Peel and slice your onions into 2 cm thick chunks. In a small baking tray (just a little larger than the size of the pork is best) arrange onions garlic and celery into a trivet for the pork to sit on. Place the pork on top of the vegetables. Add a cup or two of water in the tray (just enough to make a 1 cm layer over the base of the pan)

Place in the oven for 4–5 hours. Make a gravy with the pan juices, using a little corn-starch mixed in 1 tbsp of water to thicken the gravy—this is not technically keto. A keto friendly option is a little xanthan gum.

BOLOGNESE
(can be used for moussaka, bakes and spaghetti)

Ingredients
500 g beef mince
1 tbsp olive oil
1 carrot, diced
2–3 sticks celery, diced
1 onion, diced
2 garlic cloves, finely diced
1 cup water and a beef stock cube
2–3 tbsp tomato paste
1 tbsp dried herbs (oregano works well or mixed herbs)
1 can sugar-free chopped tomatoes
salt and pepper to taste

Method
Sauté diced vegetables in olive, except garlic, until golden brown. Add garlic and toast quickly. You can smell garlic when its cooked. Add and brown mince meat. Once all browned, add tomato paste and mixed herbs. Combine and cook for a few minutes. Add can of tomatoes then a can of water. Bring to a medium simmer. Cover and cook for 30–45 minutes *minimum*. The longer the better. Stir every 10 or so minutes and adjust heat. Take lid off for the remaining 15 minutes until sauce thickens. Serve with zoodles, cabbage noodles, or over cauli rice or konjac noodles.

MOUSSAKA

Meat ingredients above from bolognese, plus:
1 tsp ground coriander
1 tsp ground cumin
1 tsp ground paprika
1–2 large eggplants
2–4 tbsp olive oil
salt

TOPPING
¾ cup full fat plain Greek yogurt
½ cup smooth ricotta
2 large eggs
1 cup grated cheese of your choice

Use the mince recipe above and when cooking the onion, add:

1 tsp ground coriander
1 tsp ground cumin
1 tsp ground paprika

Then resume the above recipe.

Preheat oven to 180°C. While mince is cooking, fry off 1–2cm thick slices of eggplant in a shallow pan in heated oil. Sprinkle with salt. Once soft, arrange in a large baking dish approximately 20 x 30cm. Once the meat is done, layer over the top of the eggplant.

In a medium bowl, combine eggs, yoghurt and ricotta. Layer over meat. Sprinkle cheese on top and bake for 40 minutes. Allow to cool slightly before serving. Be careful! *Very* hot!

SLOW COOKER MEAT

Ingredients
500 g chuck steak (or any cheap cut of meat you like)
1 onion, peeled and roughly diced
1 carrot, roughly chopped
2–3 sticks celery, roughly chopped
1 tbsp herbs
1-2 bay leaves
1 can tomatoes
2–3 tbsp tomato paste
1 stock cube
salt and pepper

Method
Put your slow cooker on the brown or sauté mode and fry off your chopped vegetables. Brown the meat and cover in a sprinkle of salt and pepper. Add the tin of chopped tomatoes and stock cube. Set slow cooker for 8 hours on low. When it's ready, take the lid off and allow your cooker to simmer, so the sauce thickens. Serve over cauliflower rice with a veggie bake or zoodles.

CREAMY SPINACHY FISH

Ingredients
3 tbsp coconut flour
$\frac{1}{3}$ tsp salt
$\frac{1}{4}$ tsp pepper
$\frac{1}{2}$ tsp paprika
4 fish fillets like snapper, cod, salmon or hoki
30 g butter
60 g butter, extra

223

3 crushed garlic cloves
300 g spinach, fresh or frozen
¾ cup of cream

Method

In a small bowl mix the flour, paprika and salt and pepper.

Dry off the fish and pat with flour mix. Heat the 30 g butter in a deep-frying pan. Fry the fillets for 2–3 minutes on either side and put on a separate plate. Melt the rest of the butter and sauté the chopped garlic until fragrant. Add the spinach and cook for 5 minutes. Stir in cream and season. Return the fish fillets to the pan and cook through. Serve hot.

CHICKEN AND BACON ROASTED ROLL UPS

Ingredients

4 chicken boneless thighs
4 long rashers of bacon, rind removed
4 tbsp cream cheese
1 tbsp olive oil
1 tsp dried thyme
½ tsp pink salt
1 tsp garlic

Method

Preheat oven to 180°C. Grease baking tray lightly. In a small bowl mix the cheese, oil, herbs, salt and garlic together.

Lay out the bacon side by side and place an open thigh on the large end of each. Divide the cheese mix evenly over the thighs. Roll the bacon over the thighs with cheese inside, place open end down into the tray. Bake for 25–30 minutes. Rest for 5 minutes.

SUPERB SAUCES

KETO FRIENDLY CHEESE SAUCE
(super versatile and one of my favourites)

Ingredients
¼ cup cream
2 tbsp butter
¼ cup cream cheese
½ cup grated cheddar or hard cheese of choice
2 tbsp water or more cream if you need to thin it down
Pinch of sea salt, if needed

Method
Place the cream and butter in a small saucepan and gently heat. Add the cheese and cream cheese. Stir until melted and bring to a simmer. Once you see bubbles, take off the heat. Mix until smooth and creamy. If you prefer a thicker sauce, cook for 3–5 more minutes while stirring. If it's too thick, add a splash of water or cream. Use this for bakes.

VINAIGRETTE

Ingredients
⅓ cup red wine vinegar
⅔ cup extra virgin olive oil
¼ tsp salt and pepper
¼ tsp fresh thyme leaves
⅛ tsp coriander seeds
1 clove garlic, peeled and crushed

Method

Mix all ingredients and pour into a recycled salad dressing bottle with squirt cap. Screw on lid and shake gently to mix. Let marinate for at least 30 minutes before serving.

MAYONNAISE

Ingredients

1 egg
1 cup light olive oil (important)
1 tbsp lemon juice
1 tsp Dijon mustard
pinch salt

Method

Break egg into the bottom of a tumbler for a stick blender being careful not to break the yolk.

Gently pour in oil over egg. Add other ingredients. Using a stick blender, position blender carefully over the whole egg yolk, so the blender's basket encloses the egg yolk.

Blend for 1–2 seconds to emulsify mayonnaise. Pull blender up through mayo to incorporate all the ingredients until a thick mayonnaise forms. Season to taste.

KETO DRESSING

Ingredients
Dijon or stone-ground mustard
organic olive oil
lemon juice
salt and pepper
garlic

Method
Mix ingredients to your taste. Typically, 1 part mustard, 4 parts oil, ½ part lemon, then spice it up.

HOME-MADE CHICKEN SEASONING

Ingredients
½ tsp paprika powder
½ tsp garlic powder
½ tsp salt
¼ tsp ground black pepper

Method
Mix and use in slow-cooker, as a poultry or meat rub.

BEAUTIFUL BREADS

CHIA BREAD

Ingredients
½ cup ground chia seeds
¼ cup coconut flour
1 tbsp onion powder
1 tbsp garlic powder
1 tsp baking powder
¼ tsp sea salt
4 eggs
½ cup olive oil

Method
Preheat oven to 160°C and line a baking sheet with baking paper.

Combine chia and coconut flours, garlic, onion powder, baking powder and salt in a small dish, mix with a spoon. In a larger bowl combine eggs and oil whisk until combined. Transfer dry ingredients to wet and stir until smooth. Drop the dough onto the prepared sheet and spread to a 2 cm thickness, no need to fill to the sides— spread evenly with the back of a spatula. Place in preheated oven and bake for 20 minutes or until golden. Remove and cut into 8 squares. Serve hot with butter.

FARMHOUSE KETO BREAD

Ingredients
⅓ cup ground psyllium husk powder

1 ¼ cups almond flour

2 tsp baking powder

1 tsp sea salt

1 cup water

2 tsp cider vinegar

3 egg whites

2 tbsp sesame seeds (optional)

Method
Preheat the oven to 175°C.

Boil the water and mix dry ingredients in a large bowl.

Add vinegar and egg whites to the dry ingredients—combine well. Add boiling water while beating with a hand mixer for about 30 seconds. Don't overmix the dough—the consistency should resemble playdough. Moisten your hands with a little olive oil and shape into 6 rolls. Place on a greased baking sheet. Top with optional sesame seeds. Bake on lower rack in the oven for 50–60 minutes, depending on the size of your rolls. They're cooked when you hear a hollow sound when tapping the bottom of the bun.

Serve with butter—of course!

KETO BAGELS

Ingredients
BAGELS

1 ¾ cups mozzarella cheese

30 g cream cheese

1 ½ cups almond flour

2 tsp baking powder

1 egg

TOPPING

2 tsp flaxseed

1 tsp sesame seeds

½ tsp sea salt

¼ tsp poppy seeds

1 egg

Method

Preheat the oven to 220°C and line a large baking tray with baking paper. Place mozzarella and cream cheese in a medium, microwave-safe bowl and zap it on high for a minute. Remove and stir. Repeat in 30-second bursts until the cheese has melted and is easily combined.

In another bowl, mix the almond flour and baking powder, until well combined. Add egg and almond flour mix to the melted cheese mix. Mix well until a smooth dough forms. Kneading it on a non-stick surface helps with this process!

Divide the dough and form into bun shapes. Place on your lined baking tray. Use your thumb to push a hole through the centre of each bun and then shape it further until you have bagel shapes.

Place the seeds and seasoning for the topping mix into a small bowl and give it a quick stir to combine. Crack the second egg into a bowl and whisk until combined. Brush the top of each bagel with plenty of beaten egg and then sprinkle with the topping mixture.

Bake in the oven for 15 minutes.

KETO LAVOSH FLATBREAD

Ingredients
$\frac{1}{2}$ cup coconut flour
1 tbsp ground psyllium husk powder
$\frac{1}{4}$ cup olive oil
1 cup boiling water
$\frac{1}{2}$ cup shredded Parmesan or mozzarella cheese
$\frac{1}{2}$ tsp sea salt
$\frac{1}{4}$ tsp granulated garlic
$\frac{1}{2}$ tbsp black peppercorns
$\frac{1}{2}$ tbsp dried rosemary

Method
Preheat oven to 180°C and line a large shallow baking tray with a piece of baking paper. Whisk dry ingredients together in a mixing bowl. Add olive oil and cheese. Finally add the hot water, stirring continuously as it is added. Continue stirring until the flours have absorbed all of the water.

Flatten or roll/press out dough until it is thin and a uniform even thickness. Less than 3 mm thick is ideal. Bake for 20–25 minutes. Baking time will depend on the thickness of the dough.

231

When golden, transfer to a cooling rack, peel away the baking paper and allow to cool. Use a pizza cutter to cut the flatbread into squares. Store any leftovers in the fridge.

GLUTEN-FREE QUICKBREAD

Ingredients
60 g cream cheese
2 egg whites
2 tsp ground psyllium husk powder
$\frac{1}{2}$ cup almond flour
$\frac{1}{2}$ cup sesame seeds
$\frac{1}{4}$ cup sunflower seeds
1 $\frac{1}{2}$ tsp baking powder
2 pinches salt

Method
Preheat oven to 200°C.

Mix egg whites and cream cheese in a bowl.

Add remaining ingredients and work into the egg batter. Let rest for a few minutes.

Shape the batter into squares, one per serving. Sprinkle some extra sesame seeds on top if you like.

Bake in the oven for 10–12 minutes until golden brown.

Cheat sheets and quick reference guides

Baking substitutes

Baking powder
For every 1 tsp of baking powder combine ¼ tsp baking soda and ½ teaspoon cream of tartar. Use immediately.

Baking soda
For every ¼ tsp substitute 1 tsp baking powder.

Breadcrumbs
Use crushed pork rinds or almond meal.

Sugar
For each cup of sugar, substitute 1 cup powdered/granular erythritol or monkfruit.

Butter for baking
Coconut oil or lard replaces butter as 1:1.

Buttermilk
Try 1 cup plain yogurt (not Greek), or 1 cup full cream milk mixed with 1 tbsp vinegar or lemon juice.

Cream of tartar
For a recipe that needs beaten egg whites and cream of tartar, use ½ tsp lemon juice with the eggs to replace ¼ teaspoon cream of tartar.

Egg for baking
2 tbsp ground flax meal and 3 tbsp cold water for every 1 egg called for in the recipe. Let the mixture rest for 10 minutes before adding to the recipe.

Lemon juice
Use apple cider vinegar as a 1:1 substitute for lemon juice.

Powdered sugar
To replace ½ cup of powdered sugar, grind ½ cup granulated erythritol or monkfruit in a blender until fine. As much as needed to reach the amount in the recipe.

Chocolate
Substitute 1 tbsp unsweetened cocoa and ½ teaspoon erythritol for each 1 tbsp of semi-sweet chocolate required.

Sour cream
Use plain full fat yogurt as a 1:1 replacement.

Temperature conversion
100°C = 212°F
150°C = 203°F
180°C = 356°F
200°C = 392°F

Popular alcoholic beverages, average serving size, carb content

Beverage	Approx. Serving	Carb (grams)
Beer		
Regular beer	350 ml	13
Light beer	350 ml	5
Non-alcoholic beer	350 ml	12
Wine		
Dry white, red, rosé	100 ml	1–2
Sweet wine	100 ml	5
Wine cooler	350 ml	30
Champagne	100 ml	4
Sherry	50 ml	2
Sweet sherry, port	50 ml	7
Cordials, liqueurs	30 ml	18
Distilled spirits		
Gin, rum, vodka, whiskey, scotch,	40 ml	neg
brandy, cognac	40 ml	neg
Cocktails		
Bloody Mary	130 ml	5
Daiquiri	130 ml	10
Gin and tonic	200 ml	16
Margarita	250 ml	29
Martini	60 ml	neg
Piña colada	200 ml	32
Whiskey sour	180 ml	14
Mixers		
Non-caloric mixers (mineral water, sugar-free tonic, diet soft drinks)	all	0
Tonic water	100 ml	11
Tomato juice, Bloody Mary mix	100 ml	5
Juice (orange, grapefruit, pineapple)	100 ml	15

Appendix A

CUTTING CRAVINGS

IF YOU'RE CRAVING THIS...   **YOU PROBABLY NEED THIS**

CHOCOLATE

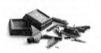

MAGNESIUM

NUTS & SEEDS

Friendly sources of magnesium include:
almonds, pumpkin seeds, green leafys,
70% plus cacao dark chocolate, avocado, seeds.

SWEET FOODS

CHROMIUM
TRYPTOPHAN
MAGNESIUM
SULPHUR

WHOLE NATURAL FOODS

Try adding foods like broccoli, chicken, eggs,
cheese, and beans - Its also worth noting how
much water you've had.

OILY OR FATTY FOODS

CALCIUM

GREENS, DAIRY

Add veggies like bok choy, broccoli or
spinach. Seafood, cheese and yogurt are also
high in these minerals. Check your water
intake.

SALTY FOODS

CHLORIDE
SODIUM

FISH, NUTS AND SEEDS

Pork crackles are a great salty high protein
food to kill the cravings. You can also head for
healthier options like roasted almonds,, seeds,
tomatoes, lettuce, celery, and olives.

BREADS, PASTA AND RICE

NITROGEN

MEAT, EGGS, DAIRY

Meat, fish, legumes, nuts, eggs, cream and
other dairy products are all high in
nitrogen.

Basic Pantry Staples

- [ ] Coconut oil
- [ ] Olive Oil
- [ ] Butter
- [ ] Himalayan Pink Salt
- [ ] Eggs
- [ ] Bacon
- [ ] 80%+ dark chocolate
- [ ] Cheese
- [ ] Pure cream
- [ ] Beef, Lamb, Chicken or Fish

- [ ] Almond flour
- [ ] Berries
- [ ] Avocado
- [ ] Erythritol
- [ ] Green Veg
- [ ] Macadamias
- [ ] Almonds
- [ ] Flaxseed
- [ ] Chia seeds
- [ ] Full Fat Greek Yogurt

- [ ] Cauliflower
- [ ] Cream Cheese
- [ ] Sour Cream
- [ ] Herbs
- [ ] Olives
- [ ] Spices
- [ ] Cinnamon
- [ ] Nutmeg
- [ ] Paprika
- [ ] Unsweetened Nut milks

Notes

For a Free Printable Version of this please go to tinyurl.com/FWordPrintables

I

Basic Pantry Clean-up

Its time to toss:

☐ Vegetable Oils	☐ Ice cream	☐ Chips
☐ Seed Oils	☐ Crackers	☐ Packet bake mixes
☐ Dressings with sugar	☐ Sugar	☐ Wheat Flour
☐ Biscuits	☐ Cereal	☐ Packaged bars - check carb content
☐ Cookies	☐ Milk Chocolate	☐ Processed foods
☐ Bread	☐ Syrups	☐ Bread crumbs
☐ Lollies/candy	☐ Rice and Pasta	☐ Pastries
☐ Skim milk	☐ Soft drinks	☐ Starchy veg
☐ Low fat dairy	☐ Sweetened yogurt	☐ Legumes
☐ Hi carb meal replacement shakes	☐ oatmeal and porrige	☐ Sauces (check lables for sugar)

Notes

For a Free Printable Version of this please go to tinyurl.com/FWordPrintables

Enjoy:

PROTEIN

- beef
- deli meats*
- eggs
- game
- lamb
- jerky*
- poultry
- pork
- sausages*
- seafood
- tofu, tempeh

FULL FAT DAIRY
- butter
- cheeses of all kinds
- cottage cheese
- cream cheese
- ghee
- heavy cream
- mascarpone
- ricotta
- sour cream
- yogurt — plain, full-fat

DRINKS
- Water:
- Still or sparkling
- water, with a spring of mint or slice of lemon or lime.
- Coffee and tea: with a little cream, if you prefer

VEGETABLES

- radishes
- rhubarb
- shallots
- snow peas
- sprouts
- herbs
- leafy greens
- leeks
- mushrooms
- okra peas
- olives
- onions
- peppers
- pickles*
- garlic
- tomatillos
- tomato
- turnip

- artichoke
- asparagus
- avocado
- bok choy
- broccoli
- Brussels sprouts
- cabbage
- cauliflower
- celery
- cucumber
- eggplant
- fennel
- sugar snap peas
- green beans
- hearts of palm
- pumpkin
- zucchini

NATURAL FATS

- avocado oil
- coconut milk
- coconut oil
- full-fat salad dressings*
- ghee
- lard and tallow
- mayonnaise
- nuts and nut butters
- nut oils of all types
- olive oil
- sesame oil

*no sugars or starches added

For a Free Printable Version of this please go to tinyurl.com/FWordPrintables

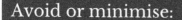

Avoid or minimise:

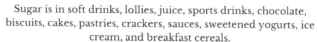

SUGAR

Sugar is in soft drinks, lollies, juice, sports drinks, chocolate, biscuits, cakes, pastries, crackers, sauces, sweetened yogurts, ice cream, and breakfast cereals.
Low-fat and fat-free milks also contain milk sugar. Sugar is hiding in many products and goes under guise of over 80 names.
Read labels carefully to avoid hidden sugars.

STARCHES

Starches including bread, cereal, pasta, rice, potatoes, French fries, potato chips, bagels, crackers, legumes (most dried beans), porridge, oatmeal, and muesli elicit a blood sugar response. Starchy foods turn into sugar when they are digested. This includes whole-grain and whole-wheat products.

FRUIT

Most fruit contains a lot of sugar. Blending or juicing isn't recommended because the fibre is important to slow blood release. Tart fruit, such as berries, lemons, and limes, or fruit with a high water content, such as melons, are do-able in moderate or small amounts.

ALCOHOL AND SWEETENERS

Some low-carb alcohols, like dry wines and spirits without sweet mixers, and low-carb beer, are fine in moderation. Diet drinks, dark chocolate, and non-caloric sweeteners can be used occasionally. The best choices for sweeteners are erythritol, monk fruit or stevia. However, some people find these, particularly alcohol, slow progress.

REPLACE

One of the most useful things you can do is to search for a low carb version of your favourite food. Do a google search and put the word keto, low sugar or low carb in front of the meal.

For a Free Printable Version of this please go to tinyurl.com/FWordPrintables

Appendix B

Tips and more recipes

www.facebook.com/TheLazyKetoMum

Even more recipes

https://tiny.one/foodweloveblog

Bio-identical ketones

Emmamartin.challenge.com

60-hour Reboot

Emmamartin.rebootnow.com

Free mini webinar

https://tinyurl.com/thefwordtipswebinar

Coaching – one on one or group

https://tinyurl.com/6weeksimple

Motivational and Educational Speaking

https://tinyurl.com/SpeakingOffers

About the author

Emma Martin was raised amidst the lush Sunshine Coast hinterland surrounded by green rolling hills and fresh seasonal food, and lives with her teenage daughter in Queensland, Australia.

With her mother being passionate about herbs and holistic healing, Emma grew up learning about many varieties of plants and seasonal produce.

Even as a child, she struggled with her weight and self worth. She excelled at writing, creative and dramatic arts and studied Performing Arts at University in Northern Queensland. There, she found herself once again feeling on the outside. After hopping from job to job, from small cruise ships through to customer service, sales and management jobs, she eventually found her feet as a bra fitter, helping other women to feel confident and valued. As she saw these women at their most vulnerable, she realised that she wasn't alone in her struggle and realised the potential for positive impact on others' lives and self-confidence.

As a mother, and particularly after her pregnancy, Emma continued to struggle with her weight. She stumbled headfirst into the keto and low-carb community, whose enthusiasm for educating what they had discovered, matched her own passion for helping others. Many were seeing extraordinary results themselves—and she leapt in! Her own resulting fat loss and extraordinary experience sparked an intrigue in nutrition and was a catalyst for her completing a Diploma of Nutrition in 2020 and becoming a certified Keto Coach in 2021. Emma is extremely passionate about exposing the many mistruths and myths, particularly around diets, diet fads and dietary fats. With her knowledge, enthusiasm and empathy, Emma spends her time coaching others and helping them achieve the same results she has had. She is excited that so many will never have to follow (or fall off) another diet *ever* again.

Resources and references

1. Davis, L. Is This Any Way to Lose Weight? *Readers Digest* [online ed]. http://garytaubes.com/wp-content/uploads/2012/02/WWGF-Readers-Digest-feature-Feb-2011.pdf

2. 69 Weight-Loss Quotes from The Obesity Code By Jason Fung. *Best Book Quotes.* http://bestbookquotes.blogspot.com/2018/08/69-weight-loss-quotes-from-obesity-code.html

3. Lilianne R. Mujica-Parodia, Anar Amgalanb, Syed Fahad Sultane, Botond Antala, Xiaofei Sune, Steven Skienae, Andrew Lithena, Noor Adraa, Eva-Maria Rataid, Corey Weistuchb, Sindhuja Tirumalai Govindarajana, Helmut H. Streya,b, Ken A. Dillb, Steven M. Stufflebeam, Richard L. Veechg, and Kieran Clarkeh. (2020). Diet modulates brain network stability, a biomarker for brain aging, in young adults. *Proc Natl Acad Sci U S A.* https://www.pnas.org/content/pnas/early/2020/03/02/1913042117.full.pdf

4. Lilianne R Mujica-Parodi, Anar Amgalan, Syed Fahad Sultan, Botond Antal, Xiaofei Sun, Steven Skiena, Andrew Lithen, Noor Adra, Eva-Maria Ratai, Corey Weistuch, Sindhuja Tirumalai Govindarajan, Helmut H Strey, Ken A Dill, Steven M Stufflebeam, Richard L Veech, Kieran Clarke. (2020). Diet modulates brain network stability, a biomarker for brain aging, in young adults. *Proc Natl Acad Sci U S A.* 17;117(11):6170-6177. https://pubmed.ncbi.nlm.nih.gov/32127481/

5. Christopher E Ramsden, Daisy Zamora, Sharon Majchrzak-Hong, Keturah R Faurot, Steven K Broste, Robert P Frantz, John M Davis, Amit Ringel, Chirayath M Suchindran, Joseph R Hibbeln. (2016). Re-evaluation of the traditional diet-heart hypothesis: analysis of recovered data from Minnesota Coronary Experiment (1968-73). *BMJ.* 12;353:i1246. https://www.ncbi.nlm.nih.gov/pubmed/27071971

5. Stephen C. Cunnane, Alexandre Courchesne-Loyer, Camille Vandenberghe, Valérie St-Pierre, Mélanie Fortier, Marie Hennebelle, Etienne Croteau, Christian Bocti, Tamas Fulop, and Christian-Alexandre Castellano. (2016). Can Ketones Help Rescue Brain Fuel Supply in Later Life? Implications for Cognitive Health during Aging and the Treatment of Alzheimer's Disease. Front Mol Neurosci, 9:53. https://www.ncbi.nlm.nih.gov/pmc/articles/PMC4937039/

6. Mujica-Parodi, L. (Host). (2020, October 31). Lilianne Mujica-Parodi Talks About How Diet and Ketones Affect Brain Aging (No. 114). [Audio podcast episode]. STEM-Talk. Podcast Notes. https://podcastnotes.org/stem-talk/episode-114-lilianne-mujica-parodi-talks-about-how-diet-and-ketones-affect-brain-aging-stem-talk/

7. Prüvit Ketosis Supplements. emmamartin.pruvitnow.com

8. Phinney, Dr. S. *Nutritional Ketosis and Ketogenic Diet FAQ.* Virta Health. https://www.virtahealth.com/faq/ketosis-ketogenic-diet-faq

9. J Yerushalmy, H E Hilleboe. (1957) Fat in the diet and mortality from heart disease; a methodologic note. *N Y State J Med.* 15;57(14):2343-54. https://pubmed.ncbi.nlm.nih.gov/13441073/

10. Dinicolantonio,, J., O'Keefe, J. and Wilson, W, L. Sugar addiction: Is it real? A narrative review. (2017). *British Journal of Sports Medicine,* 52(14). https://www.respirodeporte.es/wp-content/uploads/2017/09/sugar-addiction-is-it-real-a-narrative-review.pdf

11. Heitor A., Paula Neto, Priscila Ausina, Lilian S. Gomez, João G. B. Leandro, Patricia Zancan, and Mauro Sola-Penna (2017). Effects of Food Additives on Immune Cells as Contributors to Body Weight Gain and Immune-Mediated Metabolic Dysregulation. *Front Immunol,* 8:1478. https://www.ncbi.nlm.nih.gov/pmc/articles/PMC5672138/#

12. Phinney, Dr. S. *How much sodium, potassium and magnesium should I have on a ketogenic diet?* Virta Health. https://www.virtahealth.com/faq/sodium-potassium-magnesium-ketogenic-diet

13. 997 Convention for the Nutrition Programmes Service, Food and Nutrition Division of the Food and Agriculture Organisation.

FOLLOW ME ON SOCIAL MEDIA

Recipes, Tutorials and More...

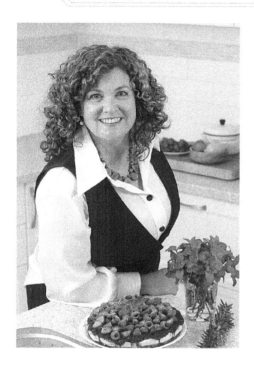

I love to share success stories, resources for inspiration and all my secrets with you!

Let's connect on social media! Be the first to hear about new recipes, tips and special offers on Facebook, Insta, Tiktok and Youtube.

Send me a message and let me know you're there.

Together we've got this.

tinyurl.com/thefwordbook

LOVE THE BOOK AND WANT M(

FREE mini-tutorial and weight loss coachiι.

tinyurl.com/thefwordtipswebinar

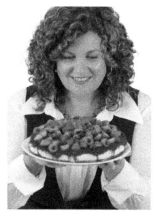

ITS TIME.

What they told us was wrong.
In a few short weeks, you can transform your jeans
size, vitality, health, sleep, energy and mood. I'd
love to invite you to join me for my mini-webinar
that will help you **never** to have to follow (and
more importantly, fall off)
another 'diet' ever.

You'll not only get exclusive access to a private
facebook group, you'll receive one on one calls,
recipes, templates, checklists, videos, cooking
classes and bucketfuls of resources and tips to help
you succeed.

FREE MINI TUTORIAL

Whether you just want to look after your
brain, age more gracefully or
lose the last 10, the free mini-tutorial I've
uploaded will help you start to make
some simple, yet impactful changes and
implement 1 degree shifts for extraordinary
success, because you deserve to succeed.

Even though fat-loss is what most of us are
seeking, this is is truly just the beginning.

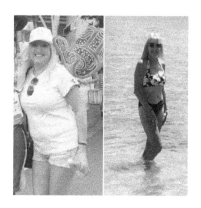

Imagine being able to fit into your favorite pair of jeans (always). Imagine
not having to dread summer and swimmers, and feeling focussed and clear
from wake up, all the way to bedtime. Imagine if you felt like a great role
model for your family and being able to not sweat the small stuff.

Imagine not being a slave to the cravings, and having the energy and
confidence to do *everything* you've always wanted to. As a side effect of
succeeding, yes - you will lose stubborn fat, however you can also improve
all of these. Imagine never having to follow another diet *ever*. Yes really.

If this sounds great to you, head on over and watch the free mini-tutorial.

Emma Martin

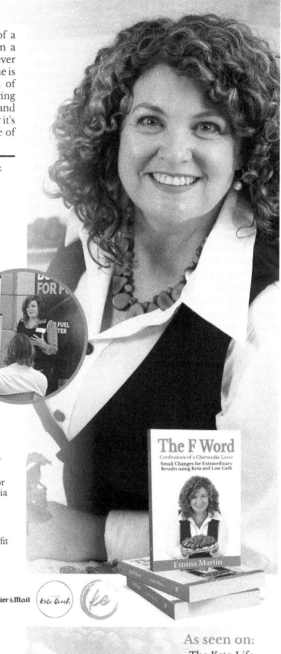

is the Author of The F Word, Confessions of a Cheesecake Lover. The book was born from a desire to help others understand how to never have to follow (or fall off) another diet, ever. She is an accredited Keto Coach, with a Diploma of Nutrition, and an accomplished and engaging Motivational Speaker. Her passion, humour, and enthusiasm fully engage an audience, whether it's 10 or 1000 people and she is already a source of inspiration to many.

Emma speaks and coaches on topics including:
* Simple steps for extraordinary results
* How to have your cake and eat it too
* Beat the guilt/repeat cycle

Why diets don't work
* How not to trip over the diet pitfalls
* Why 'energy in, energy out' is a big fat fib
* Mindset, mojo and momentum

Fat is fun
* Cooking for nutrition
* Flavour rich foods
* Simple swaps
* Feeling Fabulous

Small changes for extraordinary results
* Fat for fuel
* Banishing the inner critic
* Simple tips for success

Emma also runs #nomoredietsever workshops

To enquire about engaging Emma as a speaker for your next event or group workshop, contact her via email thefwordmatters@gmail.com or Text 0410110972 for availability and pricing.

Emma may waive her speaking fee for not for profit and causes she's committed to – just enquire

 Sunshine Coast Daily JAMES COOK UNIVERSITY AUSTRALIA  Courier Mail Keto Coach

@ emmamartin72@gmail.com
(f) www.facebook.com/emmamartinketo
www.facebook.com/TheLazyKetoMum
(www) www.ketokapers.com.au

As seen on:
The Keto Life
The Lazy Keto Mum
Intimo
Keto Transformation Workshop

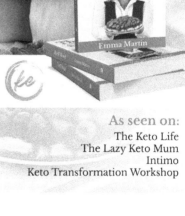

Testimonials

'This book is an eye-opening read, packed full of amazing tips, very helpful facts and insightful information.'

Nikki Monk,
Disability Support Worker

'This book will change everything you think you know about fat—compelling, funny and very insightful do yourself a favour and read it.'

Lee-Anne Johnson, Full-time Mum

'Not just another weight loss book, this is truly amazing! Emma has managed to bring science and life experiences together in one book, guiding you towards a healthy lifestyle with fantastic tips to ensure you succeed. With some simple and tasty recipes this book has everything you need to achieve your goals. Emma says it all—it's not a diet, it's a lifestyle!'

Louise Lloyd, Property Manager

'*The F Word* by Emma Martin is educational, insightful and inspiring. It's filled with proof and positivity. I now believe I *can* do this.'

Kim Davey, Business Owner

257

'I have watched Emma's growth, commitment and perseverance for over ten years. This book more than represents her and is a reflection of my own story, in the beliefs we blindly follow. I've followed Emma's journey, was sceptical, then not. She's not a megastar celebrity, she's just a mum who is dispelling those myths and presenting simple solutions.'

Carol Muir-Stokes, Travel Enthusiast, Mother and Grandmother

'Finally, an answer to why my body doesn't function well on what's supposed to be 'good for me', with all the research to back it up. Absolutely inspiring and motivating.'

Cherise Cooper, Work-From-Home Mumpreneur

'Super helpful, engaging and a fabulous read! Makes complete sense and full of incredible information to help you make clearer choices!'

Leigh Christensen, Health Administration Supervisor

'A great keto read—the recipes are simple and easy that turn out exactly like the pictures! Emma has captured all the issues we struggle with and why we often fall. A book well worth buying, especially if you love cooking and want to succeed. Looking forward to the next edition.'

Allison Mills, Registered Nurse

'This book is so informative and resonates with me. The childhood experiences mirror mine so closely. Great hints and tips to stay on track the lazy keto way. I've tried the recipes and they are easy to follow and delicious. A great guide to eating healthy and losing weight in the process. Great recipes that are delicious and easy to follow.'

Beverly Murphy, Time Poor, Busy Professional

'*The F Word* is full of so many lightbulb moments. It's an amazing read and is so helpful. It contains great research and even more amazing tips to help you succeed.'

Samantha Charlesworth,
Business Owner and Creator

'If you want guidance to a healthier lifestyle with a no-nonsense approach then this should be your go to book. Emma not only gives you the research, but in-depth knowledge on how to achieve a more energised healthy lifestyle. Also included in this book are some delicious recipes that will make you forget all about cheesecake. Enjoy.'

April Johnson, Mother,
Author and Homestead Owner

'This book is very informative and very interesting, as well as funny in parts. It certainly hits home regarding the health issues we all suffer in today's society.'

Joanne Bakos, 'Work-in-Progress'

Lightning Source UK Ltd.
Milton Keynes UK
UKHW021302230123
415821UK00021B/690